Fundamentals of
Ophthalmic Practice

A Guide for Medical Students, Ophthalmology Trainees, Nurses, Orthoptists and Optometrists

Other World Scientific Titles by the Author

Fundamentals of Glaucoma: A Guide for Ophthalmic Nurse Practitioners, Optometrists and Orthoptists
ISBN: 978-981-127-063-5
ISBN: 978-981-127-129-8 (pbk)

Fundamentals of Intravitreal Injections: A Guide for Ophthalmic Nurse Practitioners and Allied Health Professionals
ISBN: 978-981-3239-78-4
ISBN: 978-981-122-132-3 (pbk)

Intravitreal Injections: A Handbook for Ophthalmic Nurse Practitioners and Trainee Ophthalmologists
ISBN: 978-981-4571-45-6 (pbk)

Fundamentals of Ophthalmic Practice

A Guide for Medical Students, Ophthalmology Trainees, Nurses, Orthoptists and Optometrists

Tom Sherman · **William Spackman**
Southwest Peninsula Deanery, UK

Salman Waqar
Moorfields Eye Hospital, United Arab Emirates

World Scientific

NEW JERSEY · LONDON · SINGAPORE · BEIJING · SHANGHAI · HONG KONG · TAIPEI · CHENNAI · TOKYO

Published by

World Scientific Publishing Co. Pte. Ltd.
5 Toh Tuck Link, Singapore 596224
USA office: 27 Warren Street, Suite 401-402, Hackensack, NJ 07601
UK office: 57 Shelton Street, Covent Garden, London WC2H 9HE

British Library Cataloguing-in-Publication Data
A catalogue record for this book is available from the British Library.

FUNDAMENTALS OF OPHTHALMIC PRACTICE
A Guide for Medical Students, Ophthalmology Trainees, Nurses, Orthoptists and Optometrists

ISBN 978-981-127-063-5 (hardcover)
ISBN 978-981-127-129-8 (paperback)
ISBN 978-981-127-064-2 (ebook for institutions)
ISBN 978-981-127-065-9 (ebook for individuals)

For any available supplementary material, please visit
https://www.worldscientific.com/worldscibooks/10.1142/13258#t=suppl

Printed in Singapore

LIST OF CONTRIBUTORS

Mrs Sarah Levy
FRCOphth
Oculoplastics Fellow
Bristol Eye Hospital, National Health Service, United Kingdom

Miss Bryher Francis
FRCOphth
Specialist Registrar in Ophthalmology
Southwest Peninsula Deanery, National Health Service,
United Kingdom

Mr Zachary Cairns
Deputy Head of Optometry
Moorfields Eye Hospital Dubai
United Arab Emirates

Dr Rabia Salman
General Practitioner
Dubai, United Arab Emirates

FOREWORD

Fundamentals of Ophthalmic Practice is an essential read for anyone beginning their clinical journey in ophthalmology, whether as a doctor, optometrist, nurse, allied healthcare professional or student. It clearly walks the reader through the practical steps of clinical examination and investigation, preparing them for clinical life in ophthalmology. I would highly recommend this book to accompany you on your learning journey!

Dr. Louisa Wickham, FRCOphth
Medical Director and Consultant Vitreoretinal Surgeon
Moorfields Eye Hospital NHS Foundation Trust
United Kingdom

FOREWORD

Starting a career in ophthalmology can be a major source of stress for any ophthalmic healthcare provider. Starting a new position in a brand-new facility can significantly multiply the anxiety. This book provides a very important guideline for any ophthalmic practitioner. The authors have succeeded remarkably in presenting the information in a very seamless manner, where a concise medical or optical background is given, followed by a practical step-by-step description, allowing anyone to perform as a pro!

I strongly recommend this book as an essential tool for anyone starting a career as an eye care provider. It is certainly a great complement to our medical textbooks and will add very important practical knowledge in our daily practices.

Dr. Ammar Safar, MD, FACS
Chief Medical Officer
Consultant Vitreoretinal Surgeon
Moorfields Eye Hospitals
United Arab Emirates

CONTENTS

SECTION I
CLINICAL SKILLS

1

SLIT LAMP EXAMINATION

William Spackman

INTRODUCTION

The slit lamp (Figure 1.1) is the most commonly used piece of equipment in ophthalmology clinics, and being able to get the most out of it will help you accurately diagnose patients. However, it is sometimes a skill that you are just expected to pick up without any formal training. This section aims to help the reader become familiar with the slit lamp and its functions and act as an aid to learning. With practice in the clinical setting, one can quickly acquire the skills to become competent and confident using it.

BASIC OPTICS

The slit lamp bio-microscope is a compound microscope with two eyepieces mounted side by side (Figure 1.2). Each eyepiece contains two convex mirrors, which produce a vertically and horizontally inverted, virtual image. This image is then inverted by a Porro prism to produce an erect, virtual, magnified image.[1] The binocular nature of the slit lamp gives the user a stereoscopic view and allows for a detailed examination of the eye.

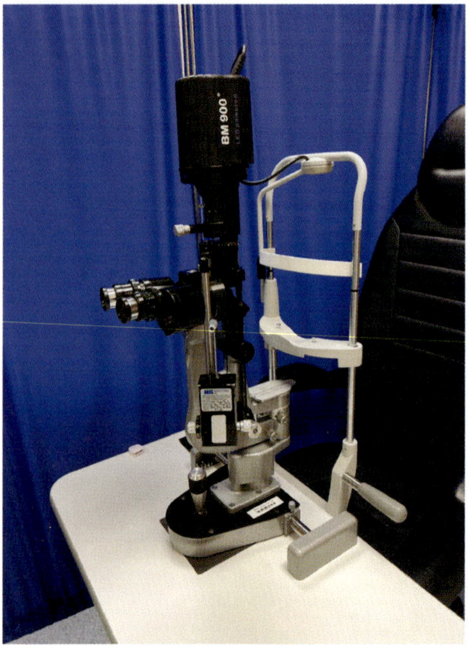

Fig. 1.1 The slit lamp bio-microscope.

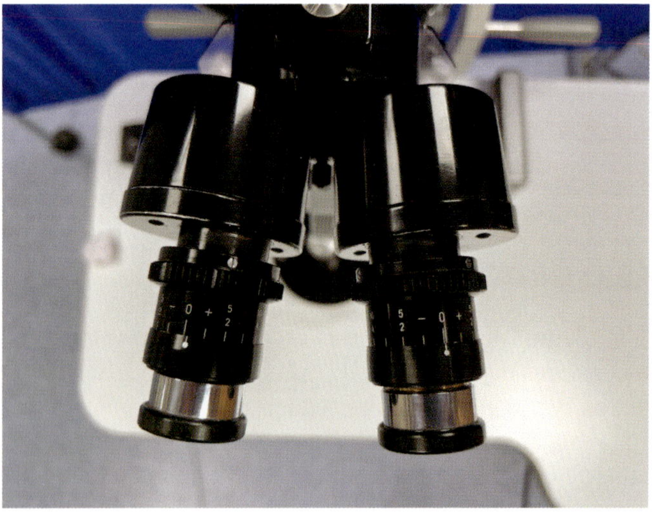

Fig. 1.2 Slit lamp eye pieces.

The working distance between the slit lamp microscope and the patient's eye is long enough to allow for different lenses or instruments to be held in this space.

Setting Up the Slit Lamp for the Examiner

Firstly, the examiner's refractive error for each eye must be dialled into each of the slit lamp eyepieces. If there is no refractive error or the user is wearing glasses, this can be left at 0. Some choose to remove their glasses for slit lamp examination and dial in their refractive error, whilst others leave their glasses on.

The examiner then needs to adjust the distance between the eyepieces according to their interpupillary distance. The eyepieces are pushed together, or pulled apart, to allow the examiner to see a binocular, stereoscopic image.

Setting Up the Slit Lamp for the Patient

Some slit lamps are at a set height and the patient's chair is adjusted accordingly. In others, the slit lamp itself is raised or lowered to the patient, and the examiner will need to adjust their own chair to an appropriate height. When adjusting the slit lamp or chair, be careful not to trap the patient's legs or arms between the chair and the slit lamp desk.

The patient's chin should be rested on the chinrest with their forehead forwards against the headrest. The chinrest can be adjusted up or down, so that the patient's eyes are aligned with the black line indicated in Figure 1.3. The patient can be instructed to hold onto the handlebars to keep themselves firmly in contact with the headrest. Correct positioning of the patient at the start will allow the examiner to move the slit lamp at will and visualise all the ocular and extraocular structures without readjusting the patient's position. This makes the examination much more efficient and comfortable. Getting into a good habit of correctly positioning the patient and examiner will save time and prevent back pain from poor posture.

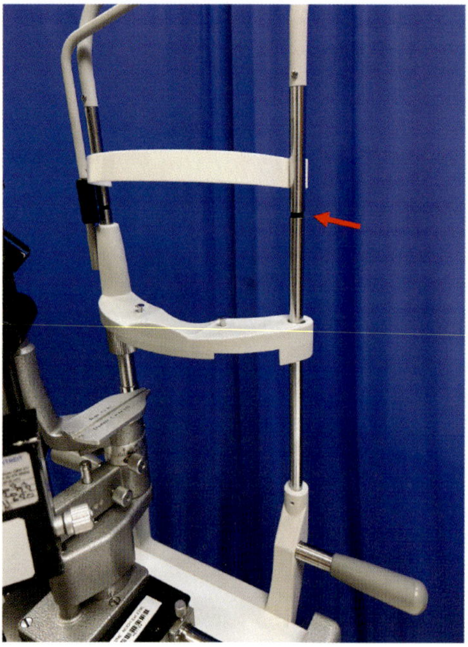

Fig. 1.3 Slit lamp chinrest and headrest for patient. Patient eye alignment guide (red arrow).

Patient Examination

Moving the Slit Lamp

The slit lamp is positioned upon a table-top and is mounted on rollers between two frames. It can be fixed to the table by tightening the screw at its base as indicated in Figure 1.4. The slit lamp can be moved up, down, left, right, forward and backward using the joystick.

The joystick is rotated clockwise to raise or anticlockwise, to lower the slit lamp. It can be moved across the table grossly

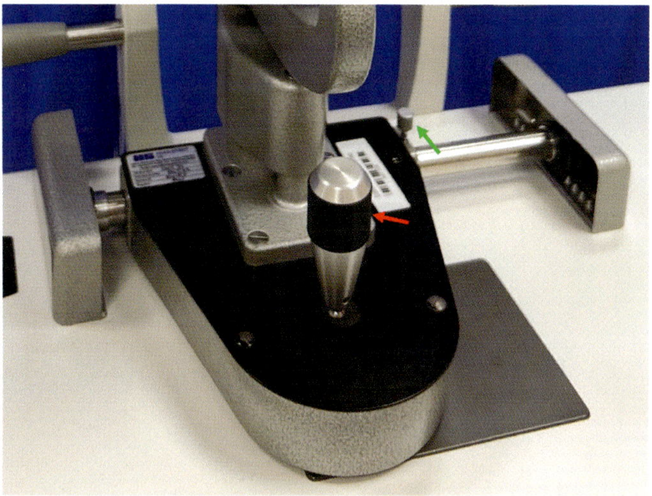

Fig. 1.4 Slit lamp joystick (red arrow). Screw to fix the slit lamp to its base (green arrow).

by pushing or pulling the whole slit lamp or finer control can be achieved by levering the joystick alone.

Turning the Slit Lamp On

The slit lamp can be turned on either by a switch or by a button, depending on its model (Figure 1.5).

Magnification

Some slit lamps have a lever to switch between low- and high-power magnification located beneath the eyepieces (Figure 1.6). Other slit lamps have a dial that can be turned to rotate through increasing powers of magnification. Higher magnification is useful to see more detail in a particular part of the eye; for

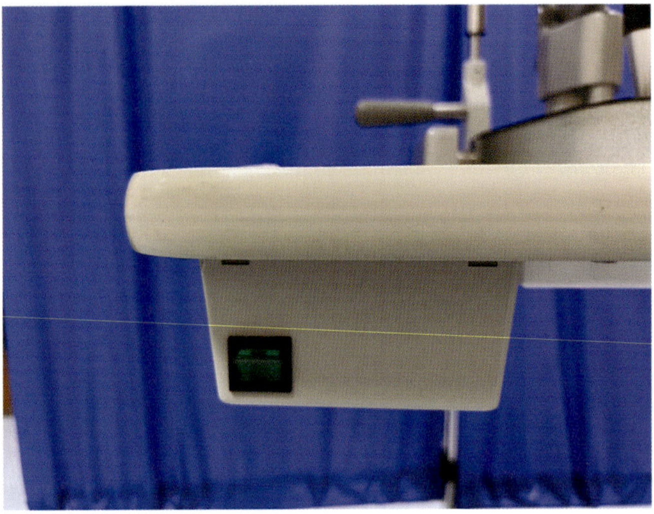

Fig. 1.5 Slit lamp on/off switch.

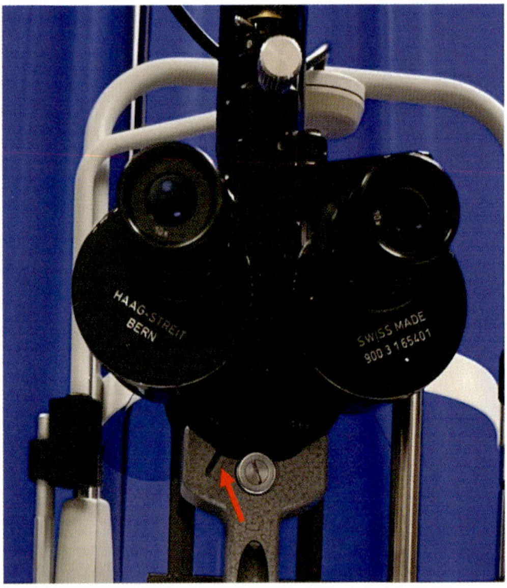

Fig. 1.6 Magnification lever.

example, when looking for cells in the anterior chamber. Higher magnification does, however, limit the field of view.

Brightness

Brightness can be changed by turning a dial on the slit lamp table or base (Figure 1.7). There may be a dimmer switch or different brightness settings to choose from. Brighter lights give better illumination but will increase photophobia for the patient. It must therefore be adjusted to the individual patient and scenario.

Filters

Various filters are used for different parts of the examination and the examiner can switch between them using a switch at the top of the slit lamp column (Figure 1.8). The furthest left setting is for unfiltered light (fine circle), then heat-filtered light (circle

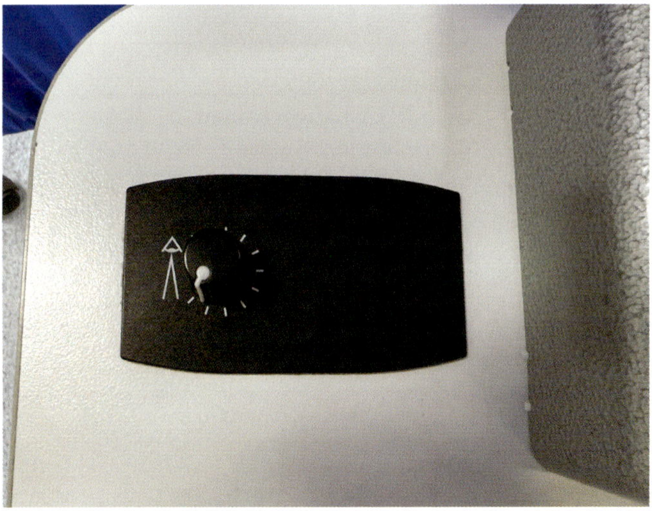

Fig. 1.7 Dimmer switch to adjust brightness.

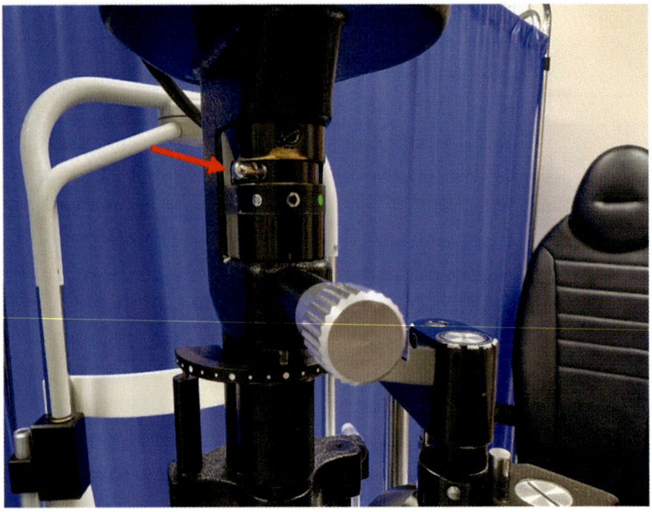

Fig. 1.8 Light filter settings: unfiltered light, heat-filtered light, neutral-density-filtered light and red-free light (left to right).

with diagonal lines), then neutral-density-filtered light (bold circle) and finally red-free light (green dot). Unfiltered light should not be used to examine the retina. The neutral-density-filtered light is less bright and tolerated better by patients. This filter should be used for retinal examination. Red-free light is useful for examining the retinal vessels as there will be greater contrast between blood, which appears black, and the retina.

Cobalt-blue light is used to identify structures that stain with fluorescein, such as corneal epithelial defects. To use this light, the silver dial located beneath the filter settings is turned anticlockwise until a blue dot appears in the window (Figure 1.9).

Changing Slit Width and Height

The silver dial (Figure 1.9) is also used to adjust the height of the slit beam. It is useful to change the height for different parts of the examination and can also be used as a measuring tool.

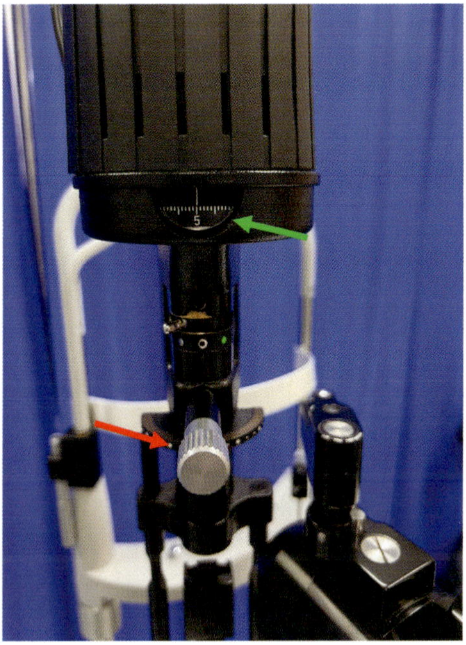

Fig. 1.9 Slit height adjustment (red arrow) and window indicating the slit height in millimetre (green arrow).

Various fixed spot sizes can also be found by turning this dial on some slit lamps.

The width of the beam can be adjusted by turning the silver dial at the bottom of the illumination arm (Figure 1.10). This can be turned to stop all light from illuminating the eye (although the bulb will still be on) and is often used to temporarily "turn off" the slit lamp.

The Illumination Column

The whole illumination column can be rotated side to side. Usually, the illumination column is coupled with the microscope so that you can see the structures that are being

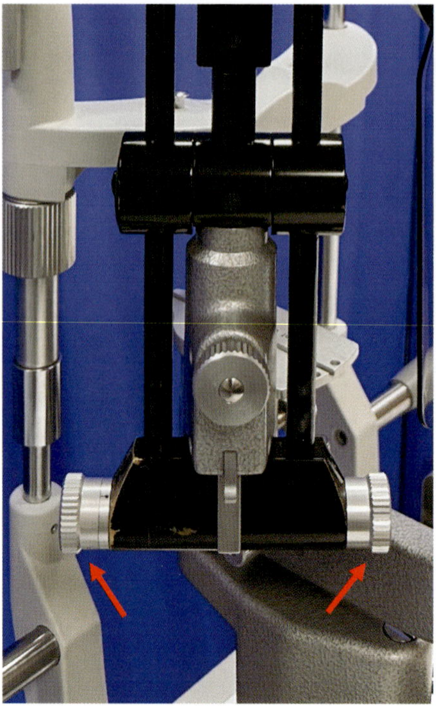

Fig. 1.10 Slit width adjustment (red arrow).

illuminated. However, the examiner may wish to uncouple the microscope and illumination column to visualise one structure whilst illuminating another. This can be done by unscrewing the silver dial in the centre at the bottom of the illumination column (Figure 1.11).

Troubleshooting

The Slit Lamp Does Not Turn On...

Firstly, check that it is plugged in at the socket, the lead is attached and it is switched on. There are different variations to

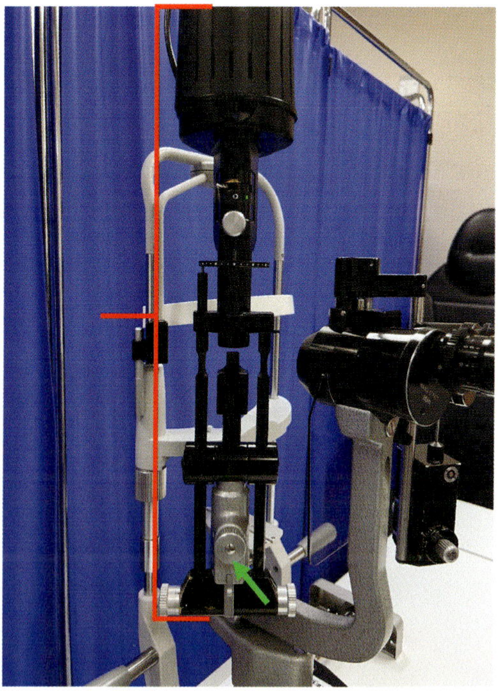

Fig. 1.11 Illumination column (red bracket), screw to couple/uncouple microscope and illumination column (green arrow).

the slit lamp, but most have an indicator light to suggest they are turned on.

Make sure that the slit width dial is turned to open the beam as this is sometimes used to temporarily "turn off" the slit beam.

If the slit lamp still does not turn on, it may be that the bulb has broken and will need to be changed. This may have occurred because the slit lamp was left on for a long time. Before changing the bulb, ensure that the slit lamp is switched off and unplugged. Each slit lamp is slightly different, but the bulb is usually located at the top of the slit lamp underneath a protective guard. The guard can be removed, and the bulb can be replaced.

Illumination Techniques[2]

Diffuse Illumination

An open beam is directed at 45° to the eye, illuminating structures that are observed directly. This allows the examiner to get an overview of the eye and adnexal structures.

Cross-Section

A thin beam is shone at 45° and the slit lamp is focused directly on the structures being illuminated. This allows for a detailed examination of the different layers of the cornea, for example.

Retroillumination

A beam is directed co-axially through the pupil to elicit a red reflex. This will reveal media opacities such as cataract, show iris transillumination and highlight peripheral iridotomies.

Sclerotic Scatter

This technique is used to observe structures not being directly illuminated by the slit lamp.

A thin tall beam of light is directed at the limbus and the light scattered across the cornea will reveal corneal opacifications.

Conical Beam

A small conical beam is shone at 45° to the eye and optics aligned so that the pupil acts as a dark background. The examiner can focus within the anterior chamber and cells or flare may be seen.

EXAMINATION OF THE FUNDUS

Learning the skill of fundal examination is challenging but it can be picked up with practice relatively quickly. To examine the retina with a slit lamp, an additional lens is required.

This is usually held by the examiner between the slit lamp and the patient's eye. There are several different lenses that can be used, each with different advantages and disadvantages, but the principles are largely the same.

It is helpful when new to fundal examination to have a systematic technique. Before long it will become second nature, like many of the techniques described above. It is best to start by examining a well-dilated eye before moving on to more challenging patients with small undilated pupils. The following is a structured method to help one achieve a fundal view:

- Dim the room lights.
- Ask the patient to look at your right ear whilst examining the right eye and vice versa. This will help keep the eye still and usually will align you with the patient's optic nerve.
- To start with, a 2 mm wide by 5 mm tall beam can be selected.
- The illuminating column must be co-axial with the eyepieces.
- Looking around the side of the slit lamp, line the beam up with the centre of the pupil and push the slit lamp as far forward as it will go towards the patient's eye.
- With your other hand, hold the lens between your thumb and index finger and rest your other three fingers against the headrest or forehead.
- Make sure that the lens is completely co-axial to the slit beam.
- When your lens and slit lamp are lined up, look down the slit lamp and slowly draw back the slit lamp in a straight line, keeping the lens completely still. The red reflex should show first and then the retina will start to come into focus.
- Identify the optic disc and macula and you can then ask the patient to look in all positions of gaze to assess the peripheral retina.
- As your skills develop, you can tilt the lens to visualise even more peripheral retina.

Fundal examination can be difficult to start with, but it will quickly get easier with practice. Being able to get a view of the retina is a rewarding hurdle to pass and will mean that you are able to examine a much greater variety of interesting pathology.

SLIT LAMP FUNDUS LENSES

A variety of different lenses can be used to examine the fundus (Figure 1.12). Fundus lenses are positive, bi-convex lenses and give an inverted view of the retina. This is important to remember when describing clinical findings. Each lens will have a different working distance. The working distance is the distance from the patient's eye at which the lens must be held to focus on the retina. This generally ranges from 7mm to 13mm.

The higher the dioptric power of the lens (d), the lower the magnification. For example, a 90d lens gives lower magnification than a 78d lens. However, the higher the magnification, the smaller the field of view. This can be overcome to some extent by increasing the physical size of the lens.

Different lenses are better for different situations. For example, when examining the optic disc or macula specifically, a lens with higher magnification such as the 78d lens might be chosen. Conversely, when examining the peripheral retina, a greater field of view is more important and a Superfield or Digital Widefield lens may be better. Most ophthalmologists

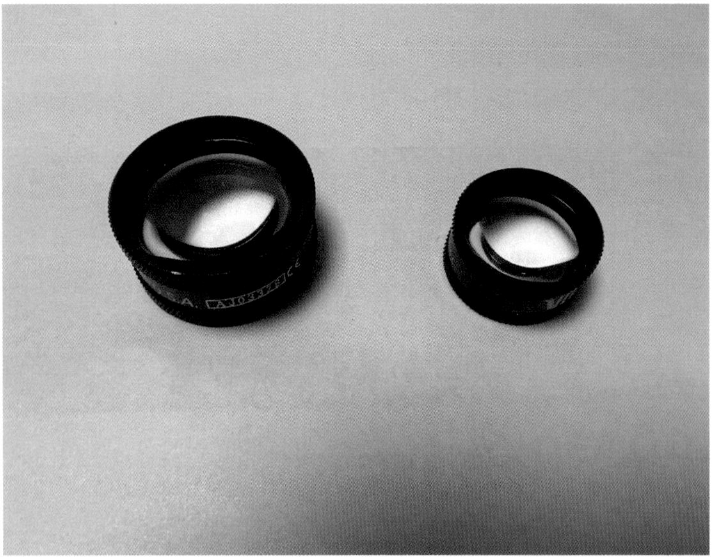

Fig. 1.12 The 78d (left) and 90d (right) are some of the most popular lenses.

will routinely use a lens with a balance of magnification and field of view. Classically, this might be a 90d or a Superfield lens. These lenses are well rounded, good for looking through small undilated pupils, and appropriate for most situations.

A summary of some of the most commonly used lenses is given below:[3]

Lens	Field of view (degrees)	Magnification	Working distance (mm)
90d	89	0.76	7
Superfield	116	0.76	7
Digital Widefield	124	0.72	5
78d	97	0.93	8
Super 66	96	1.00	11

CONTACT LENSES

Learning to use a contact lens is a useful skill. Most commonly, this is to examine the peripheral retina, the drainage angle or for laser procedures. The principles of placing the lens on the eye are largely the same and this section is aimed at achieving this.

Before placing a contact lens, the eye must be anaesthetised. This is usually done with a topical anaesthetic such as Proxymetacaine 0.5% or Oxybuprocaine 0.4%.

Some contact lenses such as the 1-mirror or 3-mirror Goldmann lens will need a viscous coupling solution applied to the lens, which will sit between the lens and the patient's cornea (Figure 1.13). This is to overcome an optical phenomenon called optical aberration. Other contact lenses such as the Posner lens do not need a coupling solution and can be directly placed on the cornea. When placing a coupling solution on the lens, it is important to ensure that there are no air bubbles as this will interfere with the view. A viscous solution such as carbomer gel 0.2% can be used.

The contact lens can be placed on the eye with the patient at the slit lamp. One technique is to ask the patient to look up and

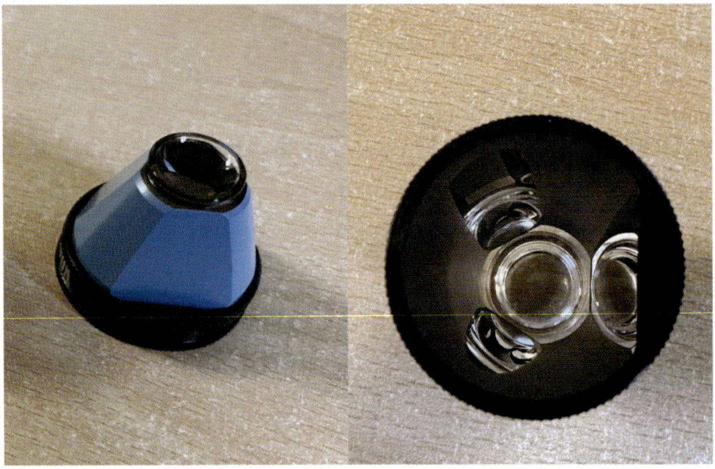

Fig. 1.13 3-Mirror fundus contact lens.

pull the lower eyelid down with your non-dominant hand. Ask the patient not to squeeze their eyes and place the lens with your dominant hand on the ocular surface inferiorly. When securely in place, ask the patient to look directly ahead and remove your non-dominant hand from the lower lid. This should align the lens directly over the cornea. The lens can then be manipulated on the surface of the eye or rotated to assess different areas of the retina or angles as required. Patients will often inadvertently pull their head back or lift their chin from the rest and so some reminders may be required. Some patients tolerate this very well, particularly those who are familiar with wearing refractive contact lenses, but others may find this quite difficult.

References

1. Madge, S.N. (2006). Clinical Techniques in Ophthalmology. Elsevier/Churchill Livingstone.
2. American Academy of Ophthalmology. (2016). How to Use a Slit Lamp. https://www.aao.org/young-ophthalmologists/yo-info/article/how-to-use-slit-lamp.
3. Gupta, A., Singh, P. and Tripathy, K. (2022). Auxiliary Lenses for Slit-Lamp Examination of the Retina. https://www.ncbi.nlm.nih.gov/books/NBK587346/

2

LID HYGIENE

William Spackman

INTRODUCTION

One of the most common clinical encounters in ophthalmology is the patient with blepharitis. First-line management is lid hygiene techniques that are taught to the patient for them to complete at home on a regular basis. It is important to be able to develop a succinct and effective way of communicating these instructions. It is also important to ensure that the patient understands why they need to perform these measures and what to expect in the natural course of the disease. This chapter introduces blepharitis as a condition and explains how to perform lid hygiene.

BLEPHARITIS

Blepharitis is by definition inflammation of the eyelids. It is very common, and some studies have shown that features of the disease are present in up to 70% of the population.[1] Some patients will be completely asymptomatic whilst others will have significant and disabling symptoms. Patients may present with a history of ocular discomfort, epiphora, photophobia or redness to the eye or eyelids. They may also describe some mild blurring of the vision and a crusty discharge from the eye in the morning.

Blepharitis is a chronic condition and symptoms will typically fluctuate over time. On examination, one can categorise the disease anatomically into anterior and posterior blepharitis although commonly they are both present together.[2] Anterior blepharitis affects the eyelid at the base of the lashes and is associated with staphylococcal bacteria found on the ocular surface. Posterior blepharitis affects the meibomian glands causing them to become dysfunctional. In anterior blepharitis, the typical findings are hard scales and crusting at the base of the lashes, which may cause adherence of the lashes to one another. In posterior blepharitis you may see oil globules at the meibomian gland orifices as well as pouting or recession. Both anterior and posterior blepharitis may cause the eyelids to be thickened and inflamed.

There are 20–30 meibomian glands in each eye lid and they secrete the outer oily layer to the tear film. This enables the tears to remain on the surface of the cornea without evaporating so easily. Blepharitis disrupts the production and distribution of this oily layer and therefore causes the eye to become dry. This may be seen clinically as a rapid tear break-up time, a frothy tear film, punctate epithelial erosions to the cornea or in severe cases, corneal ulceration. This may lead to corneal scarring and so managing these patients effectively is important.

As discussed, the first-line conservative management for blepharitis is lid hygiene and the next section discusses in detail how this is effectively performed. Other treatments may include topical lubricants for ocular surface disease or topical antibiotics if there is active folliculitis in anterior blepharitis. Oral tetracyclines have been shown to have an anti-inflammatory effect in blepharitis and a short course of topical steroid may also be used in appropriate circumstances.

LID HYGIENE MEASURES

There are different ways to perform lid hygiene and different clinicians may give different advice on how best to perform this. The following gives a guide using easily accessible equipment, which is reproducible in the patient's home.[3]

The patient will need the following:

- A bowl of clean warm water
- A clean flannel
- Cotton wool or pad
- Cotton buds or commercially available eyelid wipes

The patient can then be advised to follow the following procedures to perform warm compresses, eyelid massages and lid cleaning. These procedures should be performed in succession to each other.

Warm Eyelid Compress

Warm compresses to the eyelid help to soften the oil in the meibomian glands and allows it to pass through more easily.

1. Clean hands.
2. Soak the clean flannel in warm water and then wring it out again. The flannel should not be too hot as to burn the skin but should be sufficiently warm.

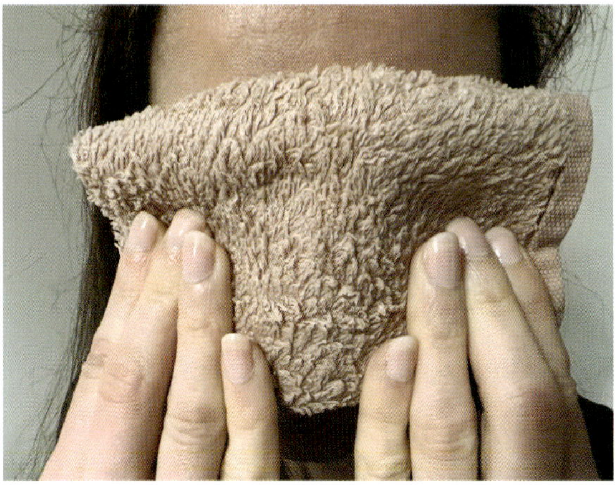

Fig. 2.1 A warm flannel is placed over the eyelids.

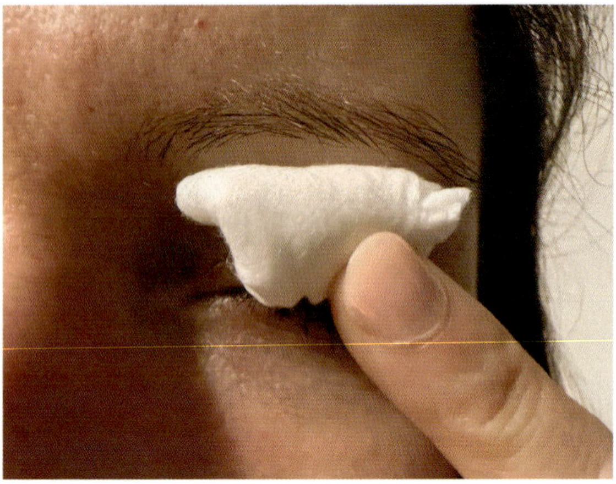

Fig. 2.2 A warm cotton pad is placed over the eyelid and massaged in a downward direction.

3. Place the warm flannel onto the closed eyelids and hold for at least 5 minutes (Figure 2.1). The water may need to be refreshed to ensure that it remains warm for the whole period.

Eyelid Massage

An eyelid massage after performing the warm compress will help encourage the softened oils within the meibomian gland to pass through the meibomian gland orifices.

1. Soak the cotton wool in a bowl of clean warm water.
2. Place the cotton wool on the upper eyelid and using your index finger, gently massage the upper eyelid through the cotton wool in a downward motion (Figure 2.2).
3. Now place the cotton wool on the lower lid and massage in an upward motion.

Eyelid Cleaning

Cleaning the eyelids will help remove crusting and excessive oils from the eyelid margin.

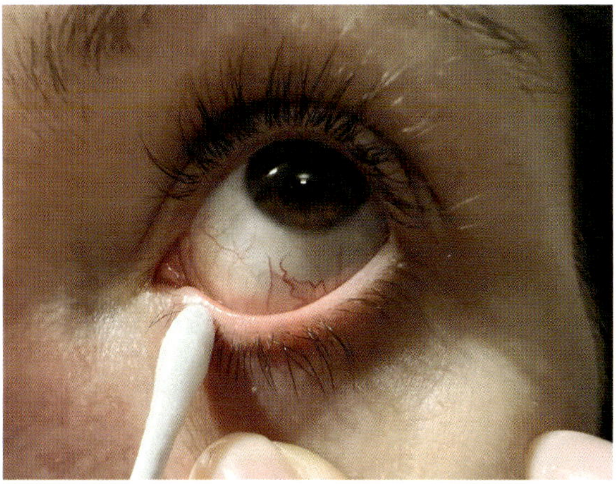

Fig. 2.3 A cotton bud is used to gently clean away debris from the meibomian gland orifices.

1. Soak the cotton bud in clean warm water.
2. Pull the lower eyelid down using the index finger of the other hand.
3. Gently clean the eyelid margin including the lashes and meibomian gland orifices just posterior to the lash line (Figure 2.3). Take care to avoid the eye itself.
4. Repeat the process on the upper lid using the index finger to hold the upper lid up.

It is helpful to appreciate that these procedures can be arduous and time consuming for the patient. It may take some patients longer than others and some may need help from relatives or carers if they are unable to do it themselves. The more the patient understands about the condition and the rationale behind the measures you are suggesting, the more likely they are to be compliant. Likening lid hygiene to brushing your teeth may be helpful in terms of establishing a daily routine.

It is important to stress to the patient that they should not expect an immediate result. Lid hygiene may need to be performed regularly over a period of weeks to months before the patient starts to notice any improvement in their symptoms.

If you do not explain this at the outset, then patients may understandably become frustrated with the lack of improvement and stop. It is also important to stress that when symptoms do start to improve, the patient should continue to perform the lid hygiene to keep the condition under control.

References

1. Schaumberg, D.A., Nichols, J.J., Papas, E.B., Tong, L., Uchino, M. and Nichols, K.K. (2011). The International Workshop on Meibomian Gland Dysfunction: Report of the Subcommittee on the Epidemiology of, and Associated Risk Factors for, MGD. Investigative Opthalmology & Visual Science, 52(4), p.1994. doi:https://doi.org/10.1167/iovs.10-6997e.
2. Bowling, B. and Kanski, J.J. (2016). Kanski's clinical ophthalmology : a systematic approach. 8th ed. Edinburgh: Elsevier.

3

LACRIMAL FUNCTION ASSESSMENT

William Spackman

INTRODUCTION

The lacrimal function test can be performed as a diagnostic and therapeutic procedure for patients with epiphora. It assesses the patency of the lacrimal system and the location of an obstruction, should one be present. The process of performing the test can also flush out debris that may be inhibiting the flow of tears through the lacrimal system and therefore improve function. This section will cover punctum dilation and lacrimal syringing.

It is important to remember the relevant anatomy of the lacrimal system as this is important whilst performing the procedure and interpreting the results. The upper and lower puncta are situated medially in the upper and lower lids.[1] The puncta open into the lacrimal canaliculi, which travel vertically for 2 mm and then horizontally and medially for 8 mm. The upper and lower canaliculi combine to form the common canaliculus, which travels medially into the lacrimal sac. The lacrimal sac is 12–15 mm in length and drains into the nasolacrimal duct which is 12–18 mm. The nasolacrimal duct opens into the inferior meatus of the nose via the valve of Hasner.

In lacrimal syringing, a lacrimal cannula is usually inserted into the lower punctum as this is more easily accessible and where most tears drain. Saline is then gently passed through the cannula and should pass through the system, into the nose and throat where it is felt and tasted by the patient. The clinician can thus determine if the system is patent under artificial, higher-pressure conditions. It is important to remember that this does not necessarily mean the system is functional under physiological conditions. Further tests with the Jones Dye Test can be helpful in determining this. If the system is obstructed, then the level of obstruction can be determined by accurate interpretation of the results of lacrimal syringing.

PRE-PROCEDURE

The procedure can be performed in the clinic setting or in theatre. To perform lacrimal dilation and syringing, you will need the following equipment:

- 2ml syringe
- Sterile normal saline
- Drawing-up syringe
- Lacrimal cannula
- Nettleship dilator (for punctal dilation)

The patient should ideally be laid back on an examination couch or reclined in a chair. There should be adequate lighting and loupes may be helpful. Ensure that the patient is comfortable and that their head is stable. A topical anaesthetic such as proxymetacaine 0.5% may also be helpful.

PROCEDURE

Punctal Dilation

It is not necessary to dilate the puncta if they are of adequate size to pass a lacrimal cannula. Punctal stenosis is present if

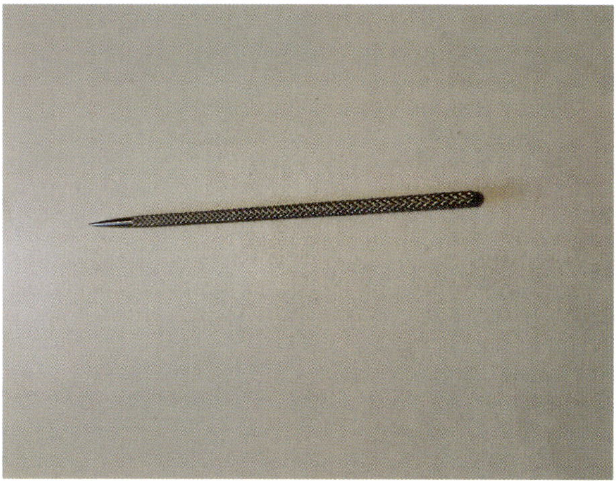

Fig. 3.1 Nettleship dilator.

they are not wide enough to pass the cannula and this is a common cause of epiphora. However, it may be helpful to establish if there is a distal obstruction in additional to punctal stenosis, as it may affect your ongoing management. Punctal dilation will allow you to pass a lacrimal cannula for lacrimal syringing in this situation.

- Pull the lower lid down and pull laterally as this will straighten the lacrimal canaliculi.
- Insert the Nettleship dilator (Figure 3.1) into the lower punctum following the anatomical direction of the lacrimal canaliculus; inferiorly for 2 mm and then turning 90° medially.
- Rotate the dilator back and forth between your thumb and index finger to help it ease into the canaliculus.
- The tapered end of the Nettleship dilator will ensure that the punctum is dilated enough to accommodate the lacrimal cannula.

Lacrimal Syringing

- Draw up 2ml of sterile normal saline into a 2ml syringe.
- Place a lacrimal cannula on the 2ml syringe and prime the cannula (Figure 3.2).

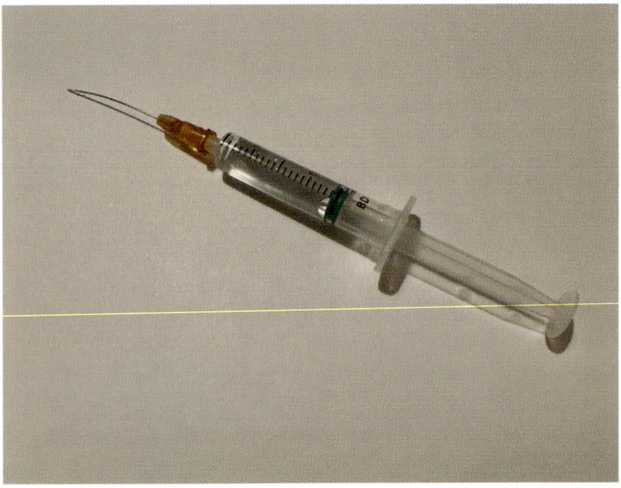

Fig. 3.2 Lacrimal cannula attached to a sterile 2 mL syringe containing normal saline.

- Pull the lower lid down and pull laterally using one hand.
- The curved nature of the lacrimal cannula allows you to orientate the cannula to follow the anatomical contours of the canaliculus.
- Insert the lacrimal cannula tip 2mm vertically into the punctum (Figure 3.3) and then rotate it within your hand to direct the cannula medially until a "stop" is felt.
  - *Be careful during this step. Glide through the canaliculus without applying pressure and if there is an obstruction, do not force the cannula through it. There is a risk of creating a false passage if this is done.*
- Take note whether the "stop" was hard or soft.
- Withdraw the cannula tip 2 mm from the point at which the stop was felt.
- Remove your hand from the patient's lower lid and use it to gently push the syringe plunger.
  - *Warn the patient and ask them to swallow and let you know if they taste salty water at the back of their throat.*
- If they do not taste the saline solution, then this indicates that there is an obstruction at some point along the lacrimal system.

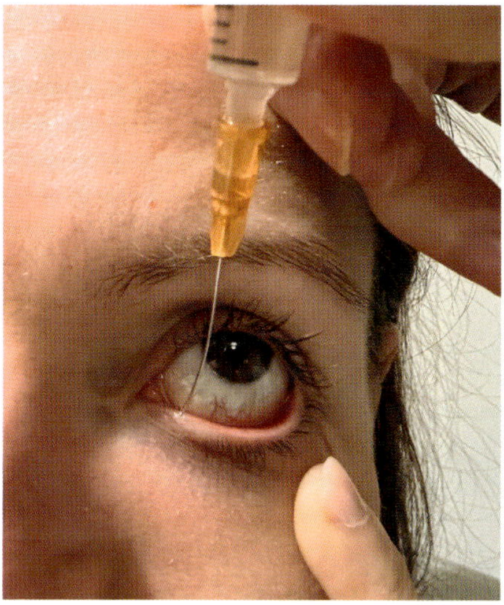

Fig. 3.3 Insertion of lacrimal syringe into inferior punctum.

- It is important to observe where the injected saline regurgitates as this will indicate where the blockage is likely to be.

Interpretation of results:

- *Saline tasted by the patient at the back of throat:* The lacrimal system is patent under artificial high-pressure conditions. This does not rule out functional obstruction and the Jones Dye Test can be performed to test further.
- *Saline regurgitates via the upper punctum*: Obstruction present in the common canaliculus or distal to this.
- *Saline regurgitates via the lower punctum:* Obstruction present in lower canaliculus.
- *Hard stop:* This is felt as a bony resistance as the lacrimal cannula has extended up to the lacrimal bone as it reaches the medial wall of the lacrimal sac. This is a normal end point and indicates the canalicular system is not obstructed.
- *Soft stop:* This is a spongy resistance and indicates an obstruction within the canalicular system.

Jones Dye Test

If the lacrimal system is patent on high-pressure testing, then the Jones Dye Test can be performed to ascertain if there is functional impairment under physiological conditions.

Primary Jones Dye Test:

- Insert a cotton bud soaked in anaesthetic into the nose on the side being tested.
- Instill a drop of fluorescein into the conjunctival sac of the eye being tested.
- After 5 minutes, remove the cotton bud.

If there is fluorescein on the cotton bud then this demonstrates function and patency of the lacrimal system. If there is no fluorescein on the cotton bud, then there is a functional obstruction somewhere within the lacrimal system and the secondary Jones Dye Test can be performed. This will help indicate where within the system there is a functional obstruction.

Secondary Jones Dye Test:

- Wash out the fluorescein from the conjunctival sac from the primary Jones Dye Test.
- Insert a cotton bud soaked in anaesthetic into the nose.
- Perform lacrimal syringing.
- Remove the cotton bud and observe if there is fluorescein present.

If there is now fluorescein on the cotton bud, this indicates there is a functional obstruction in the nasolacrimal duct specifically as the dye had reached the lacrimal sac but had not made it through to the nose.

If after lacrimal syringing there is still no fluorescein on the cotton bud, this indicates either that the punctum is stenosed or dysfunctional or that there is an obstruction within the canaliculus.

POST-PROCEDURE

Lacrimal function testing and the correct interpretation of the results will help guide further management. It is important therefore to be clear and accurate with the documentation of results.

The process of lacrimal syringing may remove debris from the lacrimal system and the patient's symptoms of epiphora may be sufficiently alleviated by this alone. If an obstruction has been identified, the patient can be counselled on the possible management options based on the level of the obstruction. This may include anything from a simple punctoplasty for punctal stenosis to dacryocystorhinostomy for lacrimal sac or nasolacrimal duct obstruction. Referral to an oculoplastic specialist would be indicated in this case.

Reference

1. Sundaram V, Barsam, A, Barker, L. and Khaw, P.T. (2016). Oxford Specialty Training: Training in Ophthalmology. Oxford: Oxford University Press.

4

PUNCTAL OCCLUSION

William Spackman

INTRODUCTION

Punctal occlusion can be performed for certain patients with dry eye syndrome. It helps by preventing or reducing the outflow of tears from the ocular surface into the lacrimal drainage system via the punctum.

The tear film is made up by the innermost mucin layer, followed by the aqueous layer and the outer lipid layer.[1] The mucin layer is secreted by goblet cells, the aqueous layer is secreted by the lacrimal gland and the lipid layer is secreted by meibomian glands. The tear film helps lubricate and protect the ocular surface whilst providing nutrition and oxygen. It also has an important role in the refraction of light. There is a constant cycle of production and drainage of tears from the eye.

Tears are drained via the lower punctum, which is located medially on the lower lid and the upper punctum which is located medially on the upper lid. The upper and lower puncta drain into the upper and lower canaliculus, respectively. These combine to form the common canaliculus. The common canaliculus drains into the lacrimal sac, which drains into the lacrimal duct and exits into the middle meatus of the nose via the nasolacrimal duct.

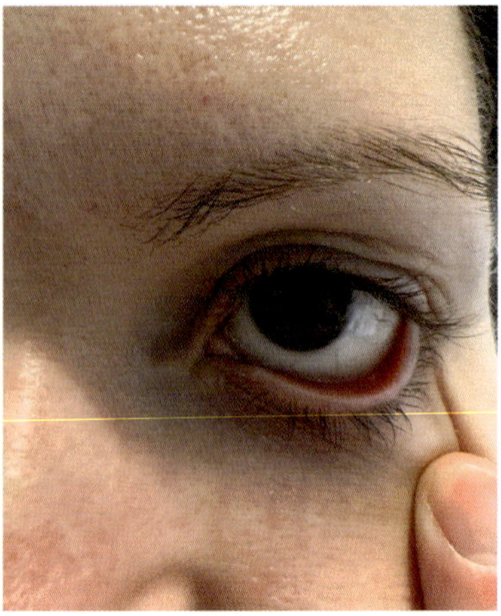

Fig. 4.1 The lower punctum is visible medially on the lower eyelid.

Through occlusion of a punctum, tear drainage is reduced, and tears are therefore maintained on the ocular surface. This can help patients with dry eye syndrome caused by aqueous tear deficiency. Punctal occlusion for dry eye caused by other mechanisms is unproven in terms of effectiveness. Patients with significant meibomian gland dysfunction may in fact get a worsening of symptoms as punctal occlusion can retain toxic secretions for longer on the corneal surface.

It is important to note that this is not first-line management for patients with dry eye syndrome caused by aqueous tear deficiency and should be reserved for patients with moderate to severe disease. Initially, alleviating environmental factors such as dry atmospheric conditions caused by air conditioning or heating systems and smoking cessation is important. Identifying whether the patient has associated systemic disease or is taking medications such as anticholinergics, diuretics or antihistamines is also relevant.

Topical preservative free artificial tear drops, gels and ointments are the mainstay of medical treatment and sufficient to control symptoms in most patients with mild disease. Topical cyclosporine 0.05% can also be used to help control the inflammatory element.

However, for patients with moderate to severe disease, punctal occlusion may be effective in managing symptoms. It can be achieved reversibly using punctal or canalicular plugs or permanently by surgically closing the punctum.

PUNCTAL AND CANALICULAR PLUGS

Punctal plugs are small silicone or collagen devices. They are usually inserted into the lower punctum (Figure 4.1) but can be placed in the upper punctum as well if necessary. Collagen plugs dissolve over a period of a few days, up to a few months, depending on the plug used. Silicon plugs will remain in place until they are removed or fall out. Some plugs are solid, whilst others will have a hole bored through to allow for some tears to drain. Canalicular plugs can also be used, and these sit deeper within the canaliculus and are not visible at the punctum.

It may be advisable to insert a punctal plug into one eye first to test its effectiveness and see if it is likely to be tolerated by the patient. A collagen plug is particularly useful as a trial plug since it will dissolve.

PRE-PROCEDURE

Most plugs come pre-packaged with an insertion device and the kit may include additional items such as a gauge to measure the size of the punctum and a punctal dilator (Figure 4.2). The insertion device helps guide the plug so that it is placed and released in the correct anatomical position. The plugs may be pre-loaded with the device or may need to be manually loaded (Figure 4.3).

The plugs need to be the correct size to ensure that they can fit within the punctum and not fall out. They should therefore fit snugly and a variety of different sizes are available to choose from.

If the punctum is too small to accommodate a plug, then a dilator may be used to enlarge the punctum. However, if there

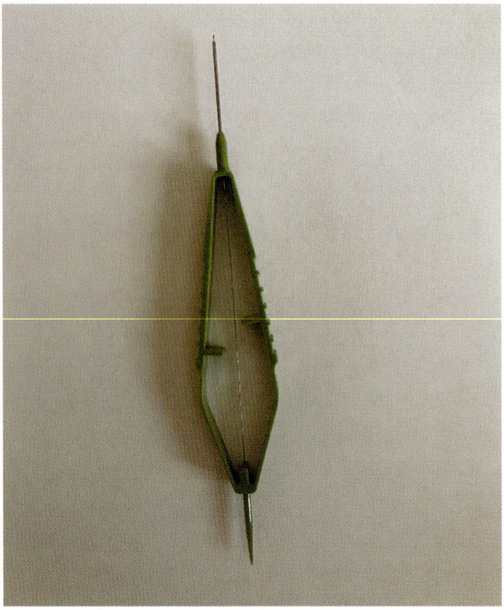

Fig. 4.2 Punctal plug insertion device with punctal dilator at one end and plug at the other.

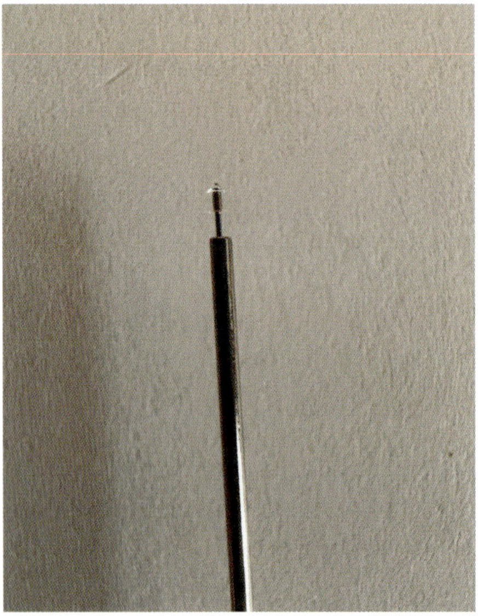

Fig. 4.3 Punctal plug loaded on device.

is punctal stenosis, then a punctal plug is unlikely to help the patient's symptoms.

PROCEDURE

- It is advisable to insert a topical anaesthetic such as proxymetacaine 0.5% in the eye to improve patient comfort during the procedure.
- The plugs can be inserted at the slit lamp to improve the view. Alternatively, you may be able to perform the procedure using loupes or simply with the naked eye. Ensure that the lighting is adequate.
- Ask the patient to look up, pull the lower eyelid down and laterally so that it is taut.
- With the other hand, hold the insertion device and place the plug vertically into the punctum (Figure 4.4).
    - Intracanalicular plugs sit beneath the plane of the punctum whilst punctal plugs should rest flush with the lid margin.
    - If no insertion device is provided with the plug, then forceps may be used instead.

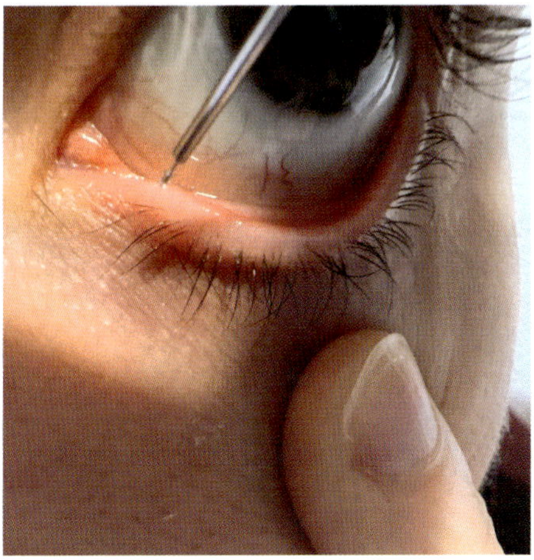

Fig. 4.4 Punctal plug insertion.

- The insertion device is squeezed to release the plug when you are sure it is in the correct position (Figure 4.5).
    - Different insertion devices will have different mechanisms so ensure to consult the product literature first.
- You can then remove the insertion device, leaving the punctal plug *in situ*.

POST-PROCEDURE

After insertion, check the punctal plug is correctly positioned at the slit lamp and that the patient is not experiencing any discomfort. Intracanalicular plugs may be seen by transilluminating the eye lid.

COMPLICATIONS

It is important that punctal plugs do not stick up and out of the punctum. They may contact the corneal surface, causing irritation, corneal abrasion and possible subsequent infection and

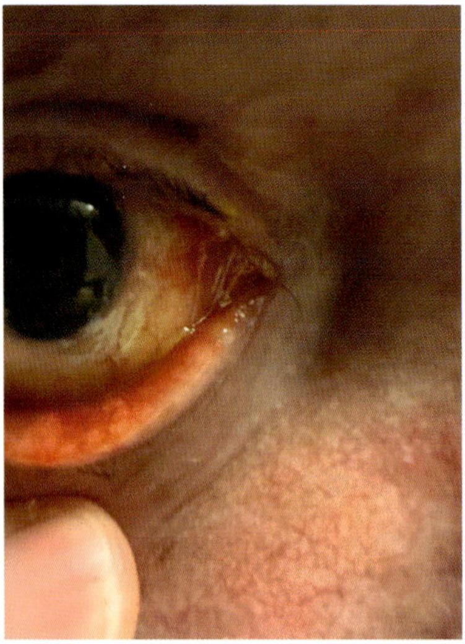

Fig. 4.5 Fitted punctal plug in lower punctum.

scarring if they do. Conversely, if punctal plugs are inserted too deeply and sit within the canaliculus, they may become stuck and require surgical removal.

Other risks of plugs include extrusion, canalicular inflammation, granuloma formation and infectious canaliculitis. The patient should be counselled on these risks and warned on symptoms to look out for.

Reference

1. Weisenthal, R.W. (2021). 2020-2021 Basic and Clinical Science Course (BCSC): External Disease And Cornea Section 8. American Academy of Ophthalmology.

5

PERFORMING A CORNEAL SCRAPE

William Spackman

INTRODUCTION

A corneal scrape is performed to detect the pathogen responsible for keratitis. Antimicrobials can then be tested in the laboratory setting to establish if the pathogen is sensitive. This will give diagnostic information and direct management in the clinical setting.

In general, a corneal scrape is recommended for lesions greater than 1 mm or if there are multiple infiltrates. A corneal scrape should be taken at presentation, prior to the initiation of any antimicrobial treatment.

A good history and examination are helpful to localise which pathogen you suspect may be causing the keratitis. This is important because you will need to send your samples on different culture media, depending on what pathogen you would like the microbiology team to investigate. Often a routine set of samples are sent to the laboratory, but you may need to send additional plates, for example if you are suspecting a fungal keratitis or *Acanthamoeba*. It is therefore important to consider what you are suspecting and know which plate to send the sample on, to clarify your clinical suspicions. A routine set may include chocolate agar, anaerobic growth agar, blood agar, Sabouraud agar and two microscope slides for Gram staining.

Particular points in the history to note include contact lens wear and if so, the type of lens being used, the cleaning regime and whether contact lenses have been worn whilst showering, swimming or in hot tubs. It is also important to establish if there has been any trauma to the eye, such as from vegetative material. The past ocular history may also help guide your clinical suspicion. Ensure that a diagram or clinical photograph is taken before the scrape for documentation and so that comparison can be made on future visits.

Local hospital guidelines will dictate the protocols you should follow but this should give a guide as to the basic principles and technique for corneal scrape.

PRE-PROCEDURE

Firstly, it is prudent to gather all your required equipment before starting the procedure. You will need:

- Topical anaesthetic such as proxymetacaine 0.5%.
- Several 21-gauge green needles (one for each sample required).
- Two microscope slides.
- Culture plates (Figure 5.1) depending on clinical suspicion:
  - Blood agar (most bacteria and fungi except *Haemophilus* and *Neisseria*).
  - Chocolate agar (fastidious bacteria, e.g. *Haemophilus* and *Neisseria*).
  - Anaerobic growth agar (anaerobic bacteria).
  - MacConkey agar (Gram-negative bacteria).
  - Sabouraud agar (fungi).
  - Non-nutrient agar with *Escherichia coli* (*Acanthamoeba*).
  - Some units may require a sterile dry swab to be sent for *Acanthamoeba* PCR testing.

Agar plates should be stored in the fridge, upside down, so that the agar is at the top and the lid is at the bottom. Check

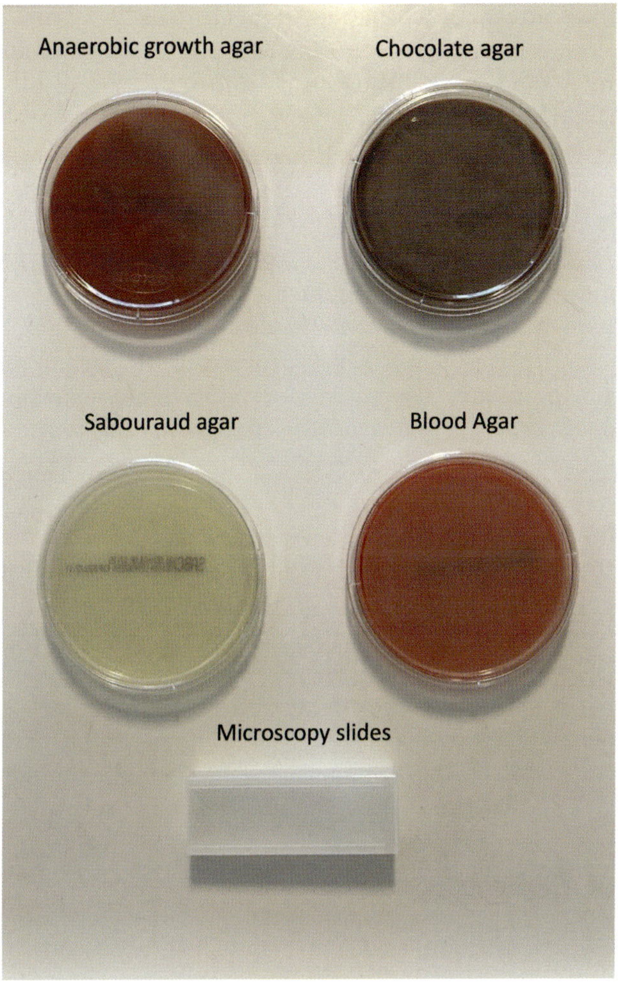

Fig. 5.1 Culture plates and microscopy slides.

there is no growth on the plates before use and keep the plates in this orientation whilst performing the scrape.

The microscope slides should be prepared by drawing a circle on the underside of the slide with a pencil which you can later place the scrape within. This helps the microbiology team to locate your sample in the laboratory.

A corneal scrape is usually performed under topical anaesthesia at the slit lamp. Rarely, it may be necessary to perform the procedure at the bedside in immobile patients, or in theatre with intravenous sedation or general anaesthesia. A discussion regarding the risks and benefits of a corneal scrape should take place with the patient.

As with any slit lamp procedure, it is important to ensure that both you and the patient are comfortable and correctly positioned. This is not only for patient comfort but also for patient safety. Typically, a needle or blade is used to scrape and an unexpected movement from the patient or clinician could inadvertently cause trauma such as globe perforation.

Instil a topical anaesthetic such as proxymetacaine 0.5%. Several drops may be required to numb the ocular surface. These patients are often in pain at baseline and adequately anaesthetising the eye is important. The more comfortable it is for the patient, the easier it will be to take a corneal scrape.

The patient can be asked to keep their eyes open or you may be able to use a spare finger to hold the upper lid whilst performing the scrape. Alternatively, a lid speculum can be used to prop the eyelids open and this may be necessary if there is excessive blinking or squeezing.

It may also be helpful to acquire the assistance of a colleague to support the patient's head at the slit lamp, so that it remains forward against the headrest.

PROCEDURE

This describes how to take a scrape using a 23-gauge green needle, although some clinicians will use a blade to take the sample.

- Align the patient's eye at the slit lamp with the area of interest in focus.
- Hold the needle in your dominant hand and approach the eye parallel to the ocular surface.
    - It may be helpful to look to the side of the slit lamp to bring your needle into the view of the slit lamp safely.

- Using the long edge of the needle bevel, scrape parallel to the corneal surface to obtain a sample from the ulcer.
  - The edge of the ulcer is most likely to contain the pathogenic microbe and so taking the sample from here is most valuable.
  - Ensure that an adequate sample is taken and collects on the end of the needle.
  - The first scrapes should be placed on the microscope slides within the circles you drew earlier.
  - Subsequent scrapes should be placed on the agar plates. Emphasis should be placed on how to plate the scrapes correctly. Generally, a series of C-shaped smears are made when depositing the corneal scrape onto the agar plates. It is important not to break the surface of the agar and so a delicate touch is required.
  - This process can be repeated to take the number of scrapes required. Ensure to use a clean needle for each scrape and safely dispose of the needles in a sharps bin.

POST-PROCEDURE

Once you have all the samples that are required, ensure that they are prepared appropriately to be sent to the laboratory. The plates and slides should all be labelled with the correct patient information, the date and time of the scrape and signed. Different departments will have different microbiology request procedures, but it is important to make sure all necessary details are completed. The site, laterality, preceding antibiotic use and clinical details should all be included. You should specifically request what tests you would like the microbiology team to perform. This is likely to include Gram staining, microscopy, culture and sensitivities. Additional tests such as *Acanthamoeba* PCR can be requested as per clinical suspicion.

If the patient has the contact lenses they have been wearing or contact lens solution available, this can also be sent to the laboratory to be investigated.

With the request form complete and samples adequately labelled, they should be sent to the laboratory as soon as possible. If there is to be a delay for any reason, then samples should be stored at room temperature rather than in the fridge.

A Gram stain and microscopy result can usually be obtained within an hour if the laboratory is contacted to request this. These early results can be helpful to direct initial management pending culture and sensitivity results, which may take several days for bacterial growth or several weeks for fungal growth.

It is helpful to draw a detailed diagram or take a clinical photograph before and after the scrape for comparison. Ensure that the patient is started on appropriate empirical treatment based on clinical suspicion and local microbiology guidelines. Arrange early, timely follow-up to assess response to treatment and act on microbiology results appropriately.

Reference

1. Weisenthal, R.W. (2021). 2020–2021 Basic and Clinical Science Course (BCSC): External Disease And Cornea Section 8. American Academy of Ophthalmology.

6

CORNEAL FOREIGN BODY REMOVAL

William Spackman

INTRODUCTION

Foreign body (FB) injuries to the eye are a common cause of presentation to A&E and eye departments. Patients will typically present with FB sensation, redness, pain, watering, blurred vision or sensitivity to light. A careful history should be taken to ascertain the mechanism of injury, the suspected FB and when it happened. These injuries are commonly acquired at work and as such, there may be medico legal implications. Thorough history, examination and documentation of findings are therefore very important. Red flags in the history should include high-velocity trauma including use of mechanical instruments, metal on metal impact such as hammering or drilling and the lack of protective eyewear. Organic material FB should also be noted as this carries a higher risk of infection to the eye.

Visual acuity should be tested and the patient thoroughly assessed using a slit lamp. The conjunctiva, fornices, everted lid and cornea should be examined for any evidence of retained FB or penetration site. Metallic FBs that have lodged in the cornea for more than a few hours will start to form a rust ring.

Fluorescein staining may be helpful in identifying FBs or entry sites. In the case of retained corneal FBs, the depth of the FB should be observed. If there is suspicion of a penetrating trauma, then a thorough examination of the anterior segment and a dilated examination of the lens, vitreous and retina should be performed. However, care should be taken not to put any pressure on the globe. Further investigation with Ultrasound B-Scan, Orbital X-Ray or thin-slice CT orbits should be considered. It is important to remember that MRI is contraindicated in the case of a metallic FB.

Deeply embedded corneal FBs may need to be removed in theatre and if there is penetration beyond the cornea, intraocular surgery will be required. This section will address superficial corneal FBs that can be removed at the slit lamp. Timely removal of these FBs can help reduce the risk of corneal compromise and maximise outcomes for the patient.

PRE-PROCEDURE

Required equipment:

- Topical anaesthetic, e.g. proxymetacaine 0.5%.
- Instrument for removal, e.g. 25-gauge needle mounted on a 5 mL syringe.

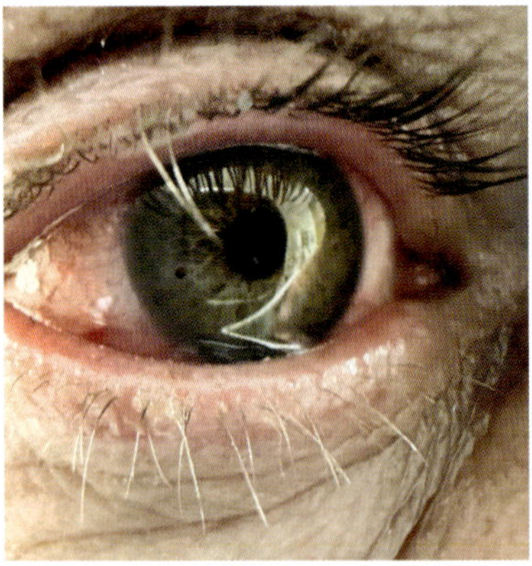

Fig. 6.1 Metallic FB embedded temporally in the cornea.

The ocular surface should be adequately anaesthetised to ensure that the patient is as comfortable as possible for the procedure. A topical anaesthetic such as proxymetacaine 0.5% can be used. The patient should be well positioned at the slit lamp, with the forehead firmly pushed against the head bar to minimise any head movement during the procedure. The patient should be advised on the importance of staying still during the procedure and should be given a fixation target in order to minimise eye movement.

Different instruments can be used to remove FBs. This can include forceps, cotton buds, hypodermic needles, magnetic instruments and mechanical burrs. Different departments will have access to different instruments and you should familiarise yourself with the available equipment. A 25-gauge needle is a useful instrument and readily available in most departments. This can be attached to a syringe to give greater support and control. One tip is to flick the bevel tip of the needle on the sheath to create a hook that can be used to remove the FB. The whole needle end can also be bent to create a better angle for access.

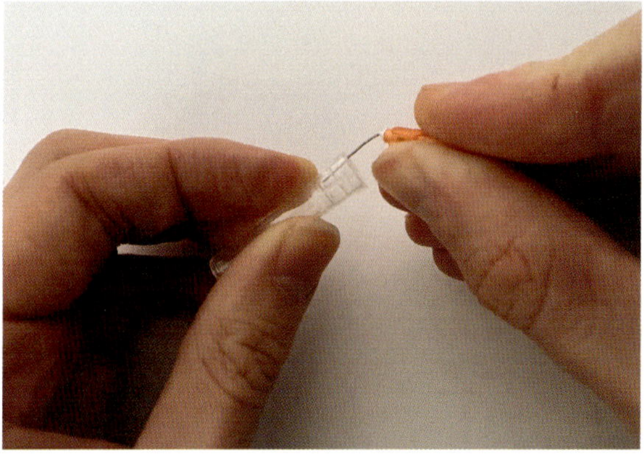

Fig. 6.2 The needle can be bent using the guard to create a better angle for removal of the FB.

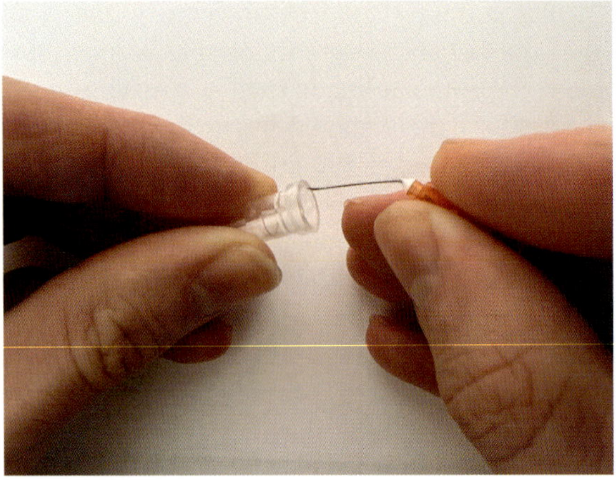

Fig. 6.3 The needle tip is "flicked" against the guard to create a small hook.

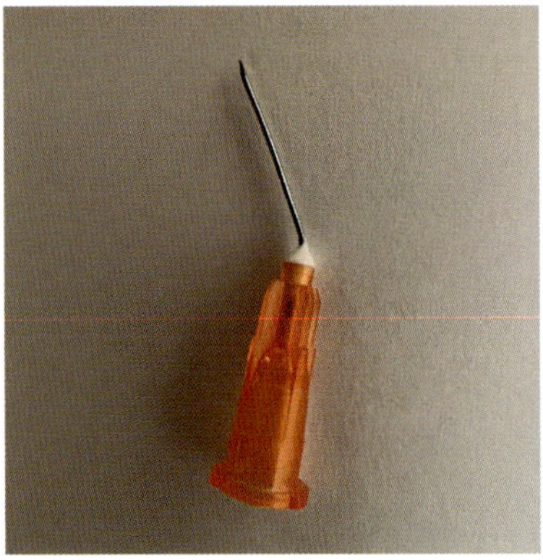

Fig. 6.4 Bent needle with small hook at the tip.

PROCEDURE

- Mount the 25G needle on a syringe.
- Prop the eyelids apart using your fingers.
- Look down the slit lamp and focus on the FB.

- Approach the cornea carefully with the bevel of the needle facing towards you. It can be helpful to look around the side of the slit lamp and bring the needle into the field of view before you look down the eyepieces.
- Carefully engage the FB at the edge with the needle parallel to the ocular surface.
- The FB should be loosened up using a gentle flicking motion. It can then be removed with the needle or with a pair of forceps.
- In the case of a rust ring created by a metallic FB, further debridement may be required. Rust rings can be removed either with a needle or with a rotating burr. Care should be taken in particular with the latter not to debride further than is necessary. In some cases, leaving the rust ring for 24–48 hours will allow it to soften and make removal easier.

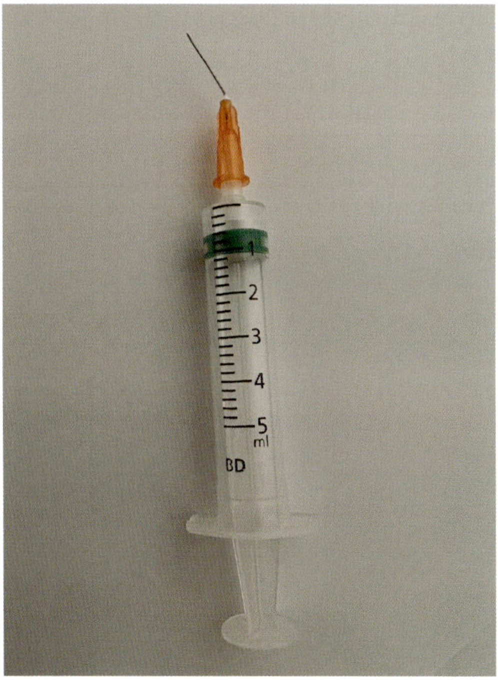

Fig. 6.5 Bent 25G needle mounted on syringe.

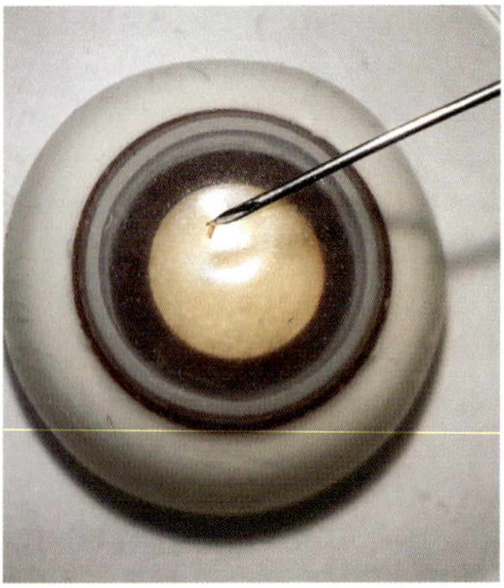

Fig. 6.6 Corneal FB removal using a needle.

POST-PROCEDURE

Once removed, the examination should be repeated to check the FB has been completely removed and that no further FBs are present. The depth of the defect should be observed and Seidel's test should be performed to ensure that there is no evidence of penetration.

A broad-spectrum topical antibiotic such as chloramphenicol ointment 1% QDS should be used to reduce the risk of infection developing and encourage the epithelium to heal. Topical cycloplegics may also be used to reduce discomfort whilst the epithelial defect heals.

Follow-up should be arranged depending on the nature and extent of the trauma and the concern regarding infection. If the FB injury was on the visual axis, scarring may affect the long-term visual outcome.

7

OCULAR IRRIGATION

William Spackman

INTRODUCTION

Chemical Injury to the eye is an ophthalmic emergency and prompt and effective irrigation of the ocular surface can help minimise the extent of damage. Severe chemical injuries can cause permanent blindness and patients presenting acutely should be seen as an emergency. Patients often present straight to the emergency department and irrigation should be performed as soon as possible. To facilitate this, various members of the multidisciplinary team will be expected to be able to perform this important procedure.

Promptness of irrigation is of upmost importance and delay for referral, detailed history or examination should be avoided. The priority is for timely and thorough irrigation, which once completed, can be followed by a detailed history and examination. Important initial history points should include what has gone into the eye, when it happened and any relevant allergies. This section aims to give a guide to the fundamentals of ocular irrigation.

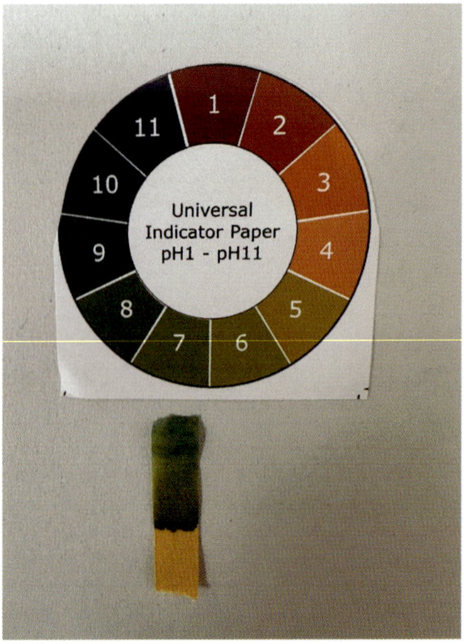

Fig. 7.1 pH paper showing a pH of 7 after being placed in the conjunctival fornix.

PRE-PROCEDURE

If readily available, it is helpful to measure the pH in the eye, prior to starting irrigation. This can help ascertain the degree of toxicity and potential for damage. In cases where an unknown substance has entered the eye, it will inform the clinician whether the substance was acidic or alkaline. The pH should be measured in both eyes using paper pH strips (Figure 7.1). This may reveal bilateral injury when the patient may think it is unilateral. If pH testing is not immediately available, irrigation should not be delayed. The normal pH of an eye is 7 with alkali substances ranging from 7 to 14 and acidic substances ranging from 1 to 7.

The patient should be positioned comfortably, ideally on a reclining chair or couch, with the head supported to minimise movement. If contact lenses are in the eye, they should be removed prior to irrigation. A drainage basin or kidney shaped bowl may be used to collect the irrigating solution as it runs out of the eye.

The patient may be in severe discomfort and plenty of topical anaesthesia is needed to facilitate irrigation. Ensuring that the eye is as comfortable as possible will help to ensure that adequate irrigation can be performed and this in turn will help maximise the outcome for the patient. Anaesthetic drops may need to be repeatedly applied during the procedure, as they are readily washed out during irrigation. Alternatively, 10ml of 1% lidocaine can be added to a litre of normal saline to produce an anaesthetising irrigation solution. This may be helpful if prolonged irrigation is required.

A lid speculum can be inserted but is not essential. Alternatively, the thumb and index finger can be used to hold the eye open as required. This also allows the clinician to evert the lid.

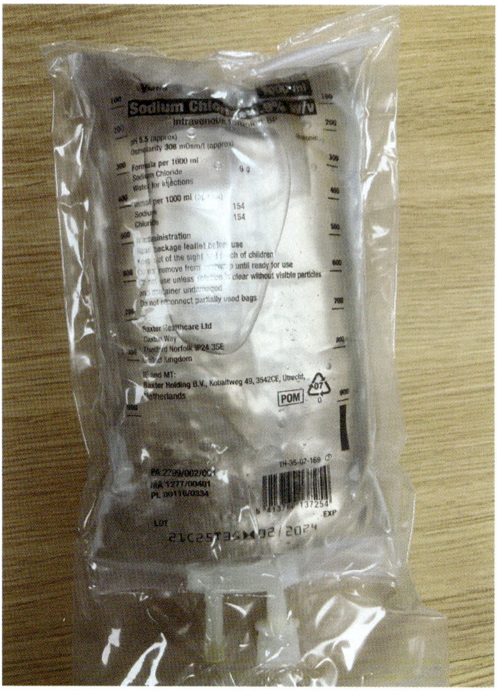

Fig. 7.2 One-litre bag of 0.9% normal saline for ocular irrigation.

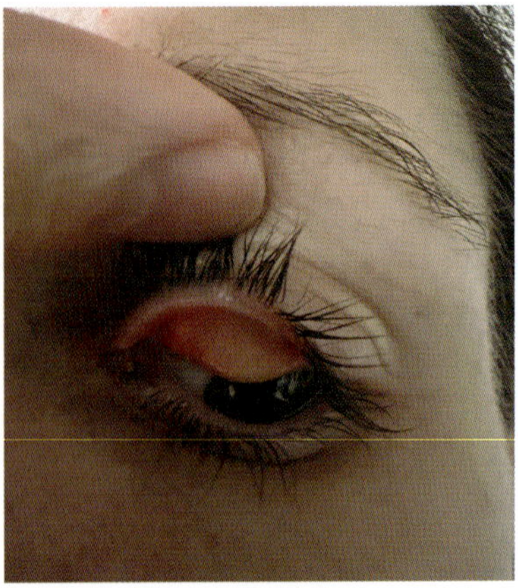

Fig. 7.3 The upper lid should be everted and irrigated.

PROCEDURE

A bag of normal saline (Figure 7.2) should be placed on a drip stand high above the patient's head, with an IV giving set attached. This will allow an adequate flow rate for irrigation. Care should be taken not to abrade the eye with the tip of the giving set.

Through the IV giving set, the entirety of the ocular surface and eyelids must be thoroughly irrigated. The patient should be asked to look in all positions of gaze. Care should be taken to irrigate the upper and lower fornices thoroughly to remove any visible and invisible particulates trapped there. The upper lid should be everted (Figure 7.3) and irrigated and then "double everted". 'Double eversion is where the upper lid is everted as normal but then lifted away from the ocular surface. This enables the full extent of the superior fornix to be irrigated and particulates can be swept away with a cotton bud.'

A minimum of 1 litre of normal saline should be used to irrigate the eye but more than this may be necessary, particularly with alkali substances such as plaster. Sometimes, several litres of irrigating solution given over several hours may be needed to completely irrigate the eye.

POST-PROCEDURE

After irrigating adequately, the pH should be re-checked. If the pH is not 7, then irrigation should be continued, and the above steps repeated, until it reads 7. Once this has been achieved, a repeat measurement should be taken 20–30 minutes later to ensure that it remains 7 and if not, irrigation should be repeated.

Once confident that all particulates have been removed and the eye is at a neutral pH, a detailed assessment can take place. A thorough history and examination needs to be performed to assess the extent of the injuries.

ASSESSMENT OF CHEMICAL INJURIES

Alkali chemicals are associated with more severe injury. This is because they are lipophilic and therefore penetrate tissues more easily. Acidic substances denature tissues, but they do not tend to penetrate so deeply.

Clinical findings to particularly look out for when assessing a chemical injury to the eye should include the following:

- Conjunctival epithelial loss
- Corneal epithelial loss
- Corneal haze, noting how clearly the iris and pupil can be seen behind the cornea
- Intraocular pressure
- Limbal ischaemia

When there is limbal ischaemia, the limbus will appear white. It is a poor prognostic sign and in the context of an ocular chemical injury, the "white eye" should raise alarm bells. A white eye may falsely reassure clinicians who are not familiar with assessing eyes, as it is counterintuitive to the usual concern that a "red-eye" brings.

Corneal epithelial stem cells arise from the palisades of Vogt at the corneal limbus.[1] These cells then slide across the cornea to repair the epithelial defect. Another role of corneal epithelial cells at the limbus is to prevent conjunctival epithelial cells from sliding across the cornea. Therefore, ischaemia at the limbus may prevent re-epithelialisation of the cornea and facilitate conjunctivalisation of the cornea, which may cause vision loss.

Another key point is to avoid being fooled by total epithelial loss. This is because you lose the contrast between intact epithelium and areas of epithelial loss. Care should be taken to avoid missing this.

It is important to thoroughly document, with drawings, the extent of trauma, so that healing can be monitored going forward. It is also important medico-legally as these patients may present from occupational trauma or assault.

The two main grading systems used in the assessment of chemical injury are the Roper Hall and Dua classifications. They are both based on assessing the severity of injury and give an indication on prognosis.

ACUTE TREATMENT OF CHEMICAL INJURIES

Chemical injuries result in significant inflammatory activity, production of free radicals and release of lytic enzymes. The acute treatment aims to address this, prevent super-added bacterial infection and promote re-epithelialisation. The following treatment may be given depending on the severity of the injury.[2]

- Chloramphenicol 0.5% preservative free
- Dexamethasone 0.1% preservative free +/– systemic steroids in severe cases
- Oral ascorbate
- Topical sodium ascorbate
- Topical sodium citrate
- Oral doxycycline

- Cyclopentolate 1% preservative free
- Preservative-free lubricants

Additional treatment options may include:

- Topical serum drops
- Conformers
- Bandage contact lenses
- Amniotic membrane graft
- Debridement of conjunctival epithelialisation of cornea

Good irrigation and initiation of the right initial treatment can have a huge impact on the outcome for the patient. Depending on the extent of the injury and healing, it may be necessary to refer these patients to a corneal specialist.

References

1. Weisenthal, R.W. (2021). 2020-2021 Basic and Clinical Science Course (BCSC): External Disease And Cornea Section 8. American Academy of Ophthalmology.
2. Chemical Injuries of the Ocular Surface. (2018). Available at: https://www.rcophth.ac.uk/wp-content/uploads/2021/01/College-News-FOCUS_April2018.pdf.

8

CORNEAL GLUING

Thomas Sherman

Corneal gluing is an important procedure to be familiar with for management of small corneal perforations. In addition, corneal glue can be applied during some elective operations on the conjunctiva to seal defects.

TYPES OF GLUE

The principal, widely available glue used for acute management of corneal perforations is cyanoacrylate glue. This is the same form of glue as commercially available superglue and glue used to repair head injuries.

The alternative form of glue is fibrin glue (trade name Tisseel, Baxter International). This is more commonly used in a theatre setting during pterygium surgery and relies on mixing two components to then produce a glue that can be used to repair conjunctival defects. As it is less widely available than cyanoacrylate glue, it tends not to be used in acute perforation settings.

Preparation of Tisseel Glue

Unlike cyanoacrylate, which is ready to use straight from the vial, Tisseel requires the mixture of components together to produce an adhesive. It uses a dual chamber syringe with fibrinogen in one chamber and a separate chamber with calcium chloride dihydrate and thrombin. When the plunger is depressed and the two syringe contents mix on the ocular surface, a seal forms.

Indications for Glue

Corneal gluing is appropriate for small perforations, usually a defect that will achieve a good result from gluing is under 3 mm in diameter. Impending defects, e.g. descemetoceles, may also require gluing to prevent a future perforation.

Corneal gluing can be performed at the slit lamp or in theatre. Corneal defects suitable for gluing at the slit lamp are usually small, central or paracentral defects without iris plugging. Where iris is plugging the defect, it may be more appropriate to repair these defects in theatre so iris can be reposited. Peripheral defects can sometimes be difficult to seal so also may be more appropriate for theatre. Where an anterior chamber is flat but the defect is small, you do not necessarily need to take the patient to theatre. The defect can be glued and the patient re-assessed in half an hour and the anterior chamber will have reformed if a sufficient seal is in place. Perforations due to infective corneal ulcers may also require some of the infected tissue to be debrided in order to make an effective seal. Cyanoacrylate glue has the advantage of being bacteriostatic to Gram-positive bacteria in this setting as well.[1]

During elective pterygium removal, allografts of conjunctiva can be sealed with fibrin glue. It can in theory be used to seal any conjunctival wound where sutures would be used, for example in strabismus surgery. However, in most cases, sutures are used in this setting. Amniotic membrane can also be secured to the ocular surface with glue.

Gluing Corneal Perforations

There are two main techniques:

1. Direct application of glue to the cornea
2. Application of a glued disc to the cornea (Figure 8.1)

General principles:

- Only a small amount of glue is needed (less than a droplet usually)
- A dry surface is needed to apply glue onto to produce an effective seal
- Dry the part of the cornea you intend to glue with the spear swab
- Always apply a bandage contact lens after the glue seal has dried as this will prevent the irregular surface of the glued area from producing pain

Direct Application of Glue to the Cornea

Required equipment: Cyanoacrylate glue, insulin syringe, speculum, spear swab, bandage contact lens, topical anaesthetic, fluorescein 2% minim.

1. Position the patient appropriately at the slit lamp or operating microscope. Usually, topical anaesthesia is sufficient (use a strong anaesthetic such as tetracaine); apply a speculum, taking care not to put any pressure on the eye.
2. Draw up the cyanoacrylate glue; an easy way to do this is by directly pushing the needle through the rounded body of the cyanoacrylate container and drawing up around 0.1 mL of glue. Alternatively, you can aspirate the glue from the spout of the container; however, this can occasionally result in a small amount of glue spilling out, which can stick to gloves.
3. Dry the area with a spear swab.

4. Using the insulin syringe, apply a small coating of glue to the affected area and allow a few seconds to dry.
5. Check the eye is Seidel negative by applying a drop of fluorescein. Wash this away once checked.
6. Place a bandage contact lens and provide antibiotic drops (usually preservative-free antibiotic such as chloramphenicol). Bandage contact lenses should be replaced every 3–4 weeks.

Application of a Glued Disc to the Cornea

Required equipment: Cyanoacrylate glue, insulin syringe, speculum, spear swab, plastic drape, punch biopsy cutter, chloramphenicol ointment, fluorescein 2% minim.

1. Apply topical anaesthetic and a speculum.
2. Use the punch cutter (should have a diameter of 2–4 mm) to create a disc out of the plastic drape (Figure 8.1A).
3. Apply a small amount of chloramphenicol to one side of the disc.
4. Draw up the cyanoacrylate glue into the insulin syringe as previously described.
5. Stick the plastic end of the spear swab to the chloramphenicol-coated side of the disc so that the disc is adhered to the swab (Figure 8.1B).
6. Coat the other side of the disc in a thin application of glue. Only a thin coating is needed and not a droplet suspended on the disc, which will be too much (Figure 8.1C).

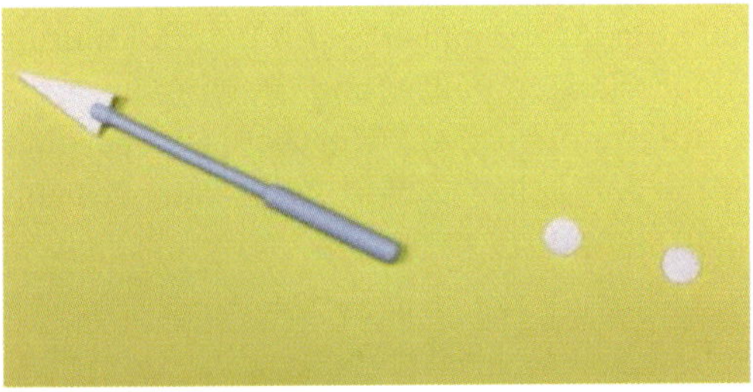

Fig. 8.1A

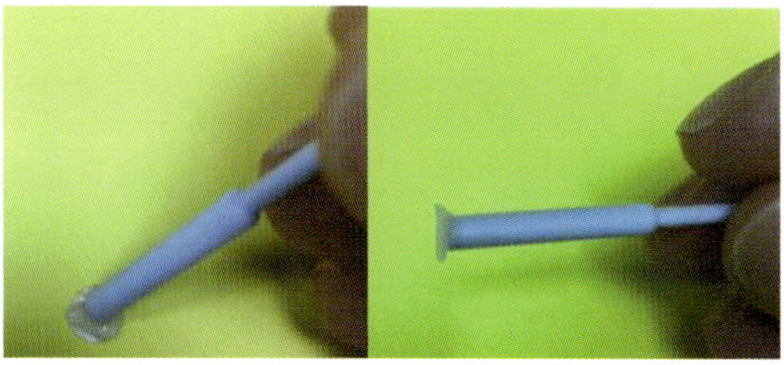

Fig. 8.1B

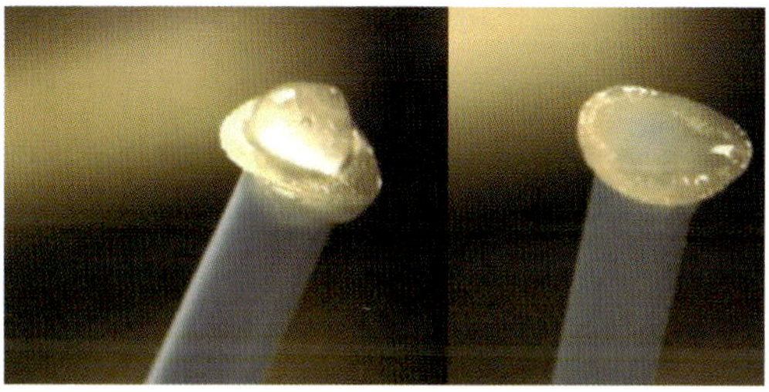

Fig. 8.1C Too much glue in left hand image. Correct glue in right hand image.

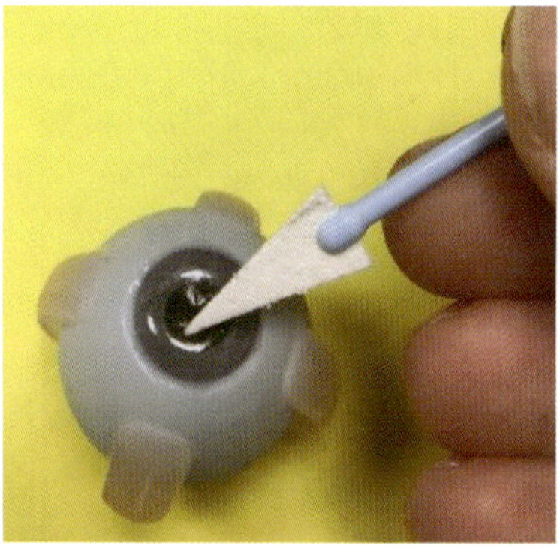

Fig. 8.1D

7. Dry the area to which the disc should be applied (Figure 8.1D).
8. Stick the disc on vertically directly onto corneal surface. Hold for a few seconds and then release, which will leave

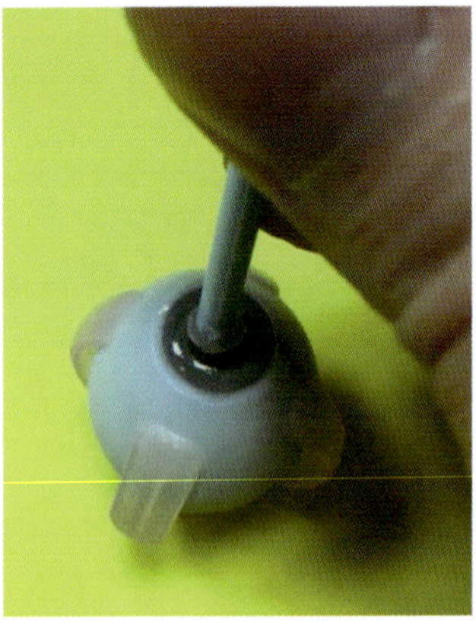

Fig. 8.1E

the disc stuck onto the corneal surface when the swab is removed (Figure 8.1E).

9. Check seal with fluorescein, irrigate and apply bandage contact lens.

It is best to review all patients requiring corneal glue the next day to ensure that the seal is still present. It is possible (although slightly tricky) to apply dilute fluorescein around the back of a contact lens by lifting the lip of the lens slightly and applying the drop. This will stain the lens but usually diluted fluorescein will wash away.

GLUING CORNEAL PERFORATION WITH IRIS PLUGGING A DEFECT

For these perforations the "double drape" technique is used.[2] This involves placing a larger diameter drape disc over a smaller diameter disc that is in direct contact with the cornea and iris tissue.

Cyanoacrylate glue is toxic to the iris so you want to avoid the iris being exposed to it. The purpose of the smaller disc is that it is applied as a glue-free patch over the iris and cornea,

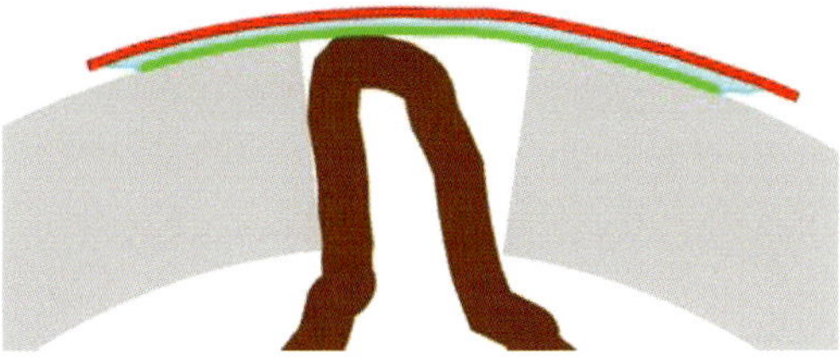

Fig. 8.2 Diagram of the double drape technique for repairing corneal perforation with iris knuckle prolapse. A larger diameter (red) disc is placed over the smaller diameter disc (green) to prevent glue coming in contact with the iris knuckle (brown).

the larger diameter disc (typically 3–4 mm in size) is then coated with glue as detailed above and applied directly over the smaller disc (Figure 8.2). Best results are achieved where any necrotic corneal tissue has been debrided beforehand. Also note that this technique is used for small "knuckles" of iris rather than larger prolapses, which will require surgical repair.

CONCLUSION

Corneal gluing is an essential procedure to be familiar with for acute corneal perforation management. The use of a glued disc is the most common technique used so is worth being particularly familiar with.

References

1. Eiferman RA, Snyder JW. (1983) Antibacterial effect of cyanoacrylate glue. *Arch Ophthalmol* **101**(6): 958–960.
2. Gandhewar J, Savant V, Prydal J, Dua H. (2013) Double drape tectonic patch with cyanoacrylate glue in the management of corneal perforation with iris incarceration. *Cornea* **32**(5): e137.

9

CONTACT LENSES

Zachary Cairns/William Spackman

The field of contact lenses has expanded rapidly over the past two decades due to new materials, designs and discovered applications. Below each lens category will be outlined along with the specific differentiating factors and uses.

INDICATIONS FOR PRESCRIBING CONTACT LENSES

Optical:
- Refractive error: anisometropia, myopia, hyperopia, regular astigmatism (sphero-cylindrical aberrations)
- Pre-refractive surgery
- Aphakia
- Keratoconus
- Corneal irregularity secondary to trauma, disease, surgery, etc.

Cosmetic:
- Iris colour alteration
- Improvement in the appearance of an unsightly eye

Therapeutic:
- Bandage lenses
- Tinted lenses for photophobia or occlusion treatment for diplopia
- Dry eyes treatments
- Ptosis prop

LENS DESIGN

The lens design refers to the shape, size, thickness and profile of the lens. These, in combination with the lens material, must allow comfort, good vision and cause no or be of minimal detriment for the wearer.

Base Curve/BOZR

Base curve — This is also known as the "Back Optic Zone Radius (BOZR)" of a lens and it refers to the primary curvature of the posterior surface over the apex of the lens.

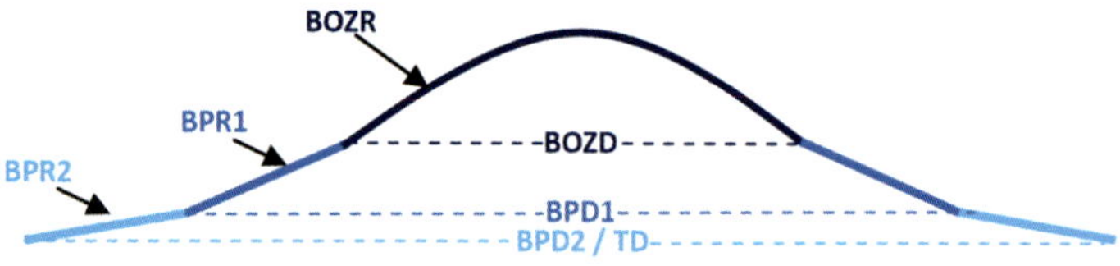

Total diameter (TD): This is the maximum diameter of the lens and will determine the overall coverage of the globe.

Contact Lens Specification

Lens: manufactures, lens type, lens code
Eye: base curve, diameter, power, lens alterations

BRIEF GUIDE TO FITTING

Basic Optical Principles

When fitting a contact lens or modifying a fitting, there is usually more than one right answer to get to a final optimum point.

A general rule to fitting: should you make a well-fitting lens bigger, you should flatten it.

To make a clinically significant change, the lens should be modified by:

— ≥0.30 mm when adjusting base curve
— ≥0.50 mm when adjusting diameter

The Basic Lens Alterations

— Every 0.1 mm BOZR = 0.5D power of the lens
— 0.5 mm diameter change = 0.30 mm BOZR change

With soft lenses usually the base curve and the diameter of the lens are already specified for optimal fitting of average keratometry values. Some manufacturers will offer two different base curve options in a specific type to aid this fitting.

APPLICATION OF BANDAGE CONTACT LENS

Introduction

A therapeutic contact lens or "bandage contact lens" (BCL) is usually a soft lens that can be applied to the anterior surface to help protect the cornea. Once inserted, the lens acts to promote healing, reduce pain, or limit the sheering forces from the eyelid during blinking. A compromised ocular surface may also benefit from reduced atmospheric exposure. The exposure is limited by maintaining contact with the cornea, thus stopping dehydration and desiccation.

Surgeries involving the corneal epithelium to be removed, such as Photorefractive Keratectomy (PRK) or corneal cross-linking, have benefitted from the use of BCLs in the recovery phase. The lens itself promotes healing by allowing the ocular surface the stability and shelter required for self-reformation. The primary purpose of the lens is to restore normal ocular function through protection, and as a result, often a low prescription or plano lens is selected. As a secondary benefit, if long-term use of the lens is required, a relevant prescription may be incorporated.

A BCL may be beneficial in a number of conditions but is most frequently used in ocular surface disease. For example, in cases of recurrent corneal erosion syndrome, the poorly adhered anterior epithelium dislodges from the basement membrane upon waking where there is a limited tear flow. Here a physical barrier between the conjunctiva and the cornea maintains stability.

Bandage lenses can also be helpful in maintaining globe integrity where corneal perforation is threatened. In this context, it may also be applied on top of corneal glue for added protection and to prevent irritation from the glue to the underside of the eyelid on blinking. This is also noted in cases of entropion or trichiasis where the short-term protection can be applied before surgical resolution.

Once inserted, the lens often remains on the ocular surface day and night for an extended period. The modality will vary according to the primary use of the lens and its approved wear schedule. Being able to insert BCLs correctly is a useful skill to acquire and may be necessary in the acute care setting.

Bandage Lens Choice

Diameter

When opting for a BCL, often the diameter is the first consideration. Depending on the site of interest, the diameter may need to be increased from the usual size of 14mm to 16 mm or even larger to achieve successful coverage. The site of interest may be beyond the cornea, i.e., a thin leaking bleb post-glaucoma surgery will require careful selection.

Lens diameter and base curve have a direct correlation to maintain a consistent fitting. As the lens diameter is increased the base curve (or steepness of the lens) should be flattened.

Material

With contact lens wear, oxygen reaches the cornea both by diffusing through the lens material and through tear exchange under the lens. The lenses should have the recommended oxygen transmissibility (Dk/t of 125×10^{-9}) or greater to reduce the risk of neovascularisation. Contraindications to extended contact lens wear include patients with collagen vascular diseases and diabetes.

Some of the more common BCLs are listed below along with the recommended replacement.

Manufacturer	Lens name	Replacement frequency
CooperVision	Biofinity	6 nights/7 days
Bausch & Lomb	PureVision 2	30 days
CIBA	Focus Night & Day	
Johnson & Johnson	Acuvue Oasys	14 days

A point to note is that continuous lens wear increases the inflammatory markers found in the tear film and increases bacterial load within the lens matrix. Usually, these levels are reduced during the lens removal and when soaking in the cleaning solution.

A patient's risk of developing infective keratitis is 10–15× greater when wearing lenses on an extended wear basis and for this reason a prophylactic (preservative free) antibiotic is recommended for cases with a disrupted epithelium.

Contact Lens Insertion and Removal

Insertion Technique

As with inserting any temporary medical device, infection control is of upmost importance. Hands should be thoroughly cleaned prior to insertion of the lens and sterile gloves may be worn to further reduce the risk of introducing microorganisms. If excessive bacterial load is present in the eye lashes this could heighten the infection risk and so blepharitis cleaning measures can run concurrently with lens wear.

Soft Lens Insertion

The contact lens will usually come in a blister pack filled with a soaking solution to maintain hydration and sterility.

1. The patient should be orientated in an upright position or lying down with the head comfortable against the headrest. Usually, anaesthetic is not required for this process, but some patients may find it of benefit if the experience appears daunting. If required, proxymetacaine or another preservative free topical anaesthetic should be inserted before opening the contact lens packaging.
2. The BCL should be placed on the tip of the index finger matching the patients eye you are wishing to insert the lens into. Allow any excess solution to drain at this point.

It is important to ensure that the lens is orientated correctly and this can be checked by looking at the rim of the lens. The lens will be a bowl shape to conform to the corneal surface or it will have a "lip" on the edge if it is inverted. A correctly orientated lens will, if pinched gently, show an inward crab-claw appearance.

3. After asking the patient to "look down", take control of the upper eyelid from the base of the eye lashes. A firm grip from above is required to hold open the patient's top eyelid and ensure control.

4. The middle finger on the inserting hand should be used to hold the lower eyelid.
5. The patient should be asked to gaze nasally, and the lens inserted on the exposed temporal bulbar conjunctiva.
6. The patient should be instructed to look temporally to the centre of the inserted lens. This allows the lens to conform to the cornea and settle into the correct position on the apex.
7. The eyelids can be released once the lens has taken residence.
8. If a bubble has been introduced under the lens or there is difficulty in centring the lens, ask the patient to close the eye and massage gently to settle.

Document the lens details such as lens type, base curve, diameter and power.

Soft Lens Removal

This technique is very similar to the insertion process.

1. Orientate yourself to the side of the lens being removed. As before, remove a lens from the eye with the corresponding hand, i.e., left eye with the left hand or vice versa.
2. Ask the patient to look down and take control of the upper eye lid using the non-removing hand.
3. To expose more conjunctiva and aid in lens removal, hold the lower eye lid with the removing hand (usually the middle finger).
4. Instruct the patient to look nasally and dislodge the lens onto the temporal bulbar conjunctiva.
5. Pinch the lens with the thumb and forefinger — A wide grip initially will allow the lens to wrinkle to aid in removal.

Tip — If the ocular surface is dry, the lens can appear to be adhered and so more difficult to remove. An ocular lubricating drop moments before can help with removal.

Post-Procedure Care and Complications

It is important to counsel the patient on the risks of contact lens wear, particularly in continuous wear lenses which remain in the eye for an extended period of time; 30 days continuously in some cases.

As with any contact lens, there is always a risk of introducing microorganisms to the eye, which may lead to an infectious keratitis. Encouraging good hygiene and asking the patient to avoid swimming or getting water into the eye will reduce the risk of infection.

Contact lenses may cause or exacerbate dry eye syndromes and could lead to corneal hypoxia and oedema. Counselling patients on these risks, advising them on signs and symptoms to look out for and monitoring patients wearing a BCL is important.

Lens Movement and Fitting

In a normal eye, once settled, the lens appears to remain stationary on primary gaze. Upon blinking a modern silicone hydrogel lens is expected to have some movement of <0.5 mm. This allows for tear exchange to take place under the lens with the primary purpose of removing debris. The lens is expected to rapidly relocate to the starting position post blink.

The lens may be slightly decentred below the corneal apex due to gravity. When assessing the lens, this is likely to be noted as the distance from the limbus to the lens edge will be greater if measured inferiorly. This is to be expected and deemed acceptable should all the other criteria be met.

The bandage lens is expected to give full corneal coverage and limit exposure in the site of interest if it is outside the limbus.

Common CL Issues

Although many anterior eye issues can cause contact lens complications (such as blepharitis and meibomian gland dysfunction), the following are some of the complications seen as a direct result of lens wear.

Contact Lens-Related Dryness

Even with the advancements made in contact lens materials and coatings, the most common deterrent from lens wear has consistently been ocular surface dryness, which has been exacerbated by lens wear.

This dryness is often due to lens dehydration and exacerbated by excessive wearing schedules. A movement towards silicone hydrogel materials has enabled practitioners to fit lenses with an initial lower water content and so reducing the dehydration effect experienced by the lens. Many manufacturers have taken this concept of lens dehydration further by applying coatings to mimic the ocular surface and increase wearing times.

As in the case of ocular dryness, often patients will be symptomatic of tired, gritty or dryness caused by the lens wear, and this should be addressed at the earliest stages.

On anterior eye assessment, it is common to see superficial epithelial staining of the cornea and conjunctiva, coupled with diffuse low-grade hyperaemia. Lens wear is generally well tolerated despite the clinical signs.

These patients should be moved to an improved contact lens material, advised on excessive wearing times, and recommended lubrication drops periodically through the day. If the patient has been wearing the same lens type for many years, suggest a contact lens appointment with their local optometrist to discuss some of the latest technologies and materials to improve comfort.

When adding an ocular lubricant to a patient's daily routine, it is often advised to complement it with a recurring task in their routine. An example of this is to ask the patient to insert a lubricating drop whenever they have a cup of coffee throughout the day.

Contact Lens Solution Toxicity

With all monthly replacement lenses a storage and cleaning solution is required to maintain lens hydration and act as a disinfecting agent. The solutions can contain many different molecules and preservatives which the ocular surface may be sensitive to.

If an acute issue of contact lens intolerance is experienced, a detailed history may highlight the recent change in brand or ingredients responsible. A common reporting from patients with solution toxicity is an initial irritation on lens insertion, followed by a gradual improvement throughout the day. As the solutions concentration diminishes, the eye will become more comfortable.

A conjunctival papillary response can often be noted due to the allergic nature of the solution toxicity. When examining the patient, extra care should be taken to note any papillae, mucus discharge or diffuse conjunctival hyperaemia.

The patient should be recommended to change the care systems currently used and move to a preservative-free option if available. The option of a daily disposable lens may also solve the issue as it completely removes the necessity for a supplementary solution.

10

SUTURE REMOVAL

William Spackman

INTRODUCTION

Sutures may need to be removed routinely after surgery or because a suture is causing complications. Since the sutures used in ophthalmology are very small and the tissues that they are placed in are delicate, a good technique for removal is important. The following are some of the indications for suture removal from the ocular surface:

- Removal of suture following corneal or cataract surgery.
- Removal of a releasable suture following trabeculectomy.
- To reverse astigmatism caused by a corneal suture.
- Suture is a site of infection.
- Loose sutures.
- Broken sutures.

Loose corneal sutures should be removed as they may be a site for inflammation or infection and if they are not supporting a wound, they are not offering any benefit. Likewise, broken sutures should also be removed.

PRE-PROCEDURE

Gather the equipment required for removal of the suture.

- Topical anaesthetic, e.g. proxymetacaine 0.5%
- Topical povidone-iodine 5% drops
- Orange (25-gauge) or Yellow (30-gauge) needle
- Suture removal forceps, e.g. Jewellers Forceps (Figure 10.1)
- Chloramphenicol 0.5% eye drops
- If available, the Waqar suture removal forceps (available from Beaver-Visitec International) can allow for breakage and removal of suture in one quick movement. It has a perpendicular tip incorporated into the distal end (orange arrow), which is slid under the suture to break it followed by removal with the forceps (Figure 10.3).

Firstly, instil the topical anaesthetic, followed by the povidone-iodine drops. It is advisable to remove ocular surface sutures at the slit lamp. Ensure that both yourself and the patient are comfortable at the slit lamp with the height correctly adjusted. The patient's forehead should be firmly forward against the headrest to ensure that there are no unexpected

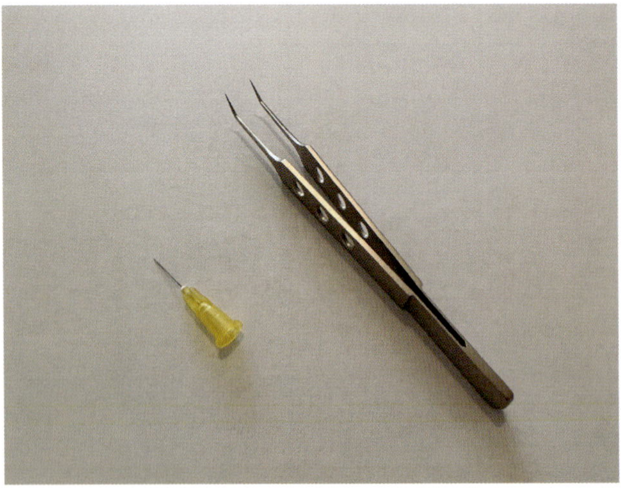

Fig. 10.1 30G needle and jewellers forceps for suture removal.

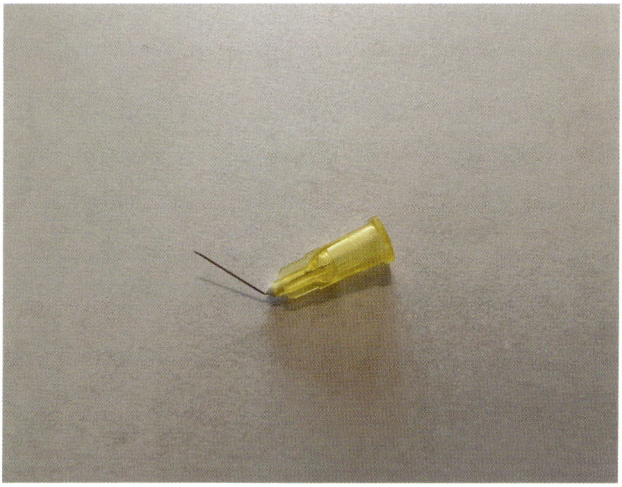

Fig. 10.2 30G needle bent to improve access to the corneal suture.

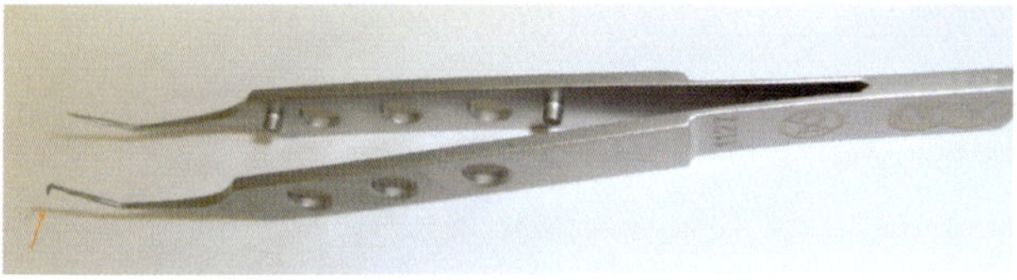

Fig. 10.3 Waqar suture removal forceps.

movements when you are removing the suture. As discussed in the foreign body removal section, it may be helpful to bend the needle to improve the angle of approach (Figure 10.2).

PROCEDURE

Use one hand to control the slit lamp and the other hand to retract the patient's upper lid and simultaneously hold the needle. It may be helpful to have the assistance of a colleague to retract the upper lid for you or use a lid speculum. Ask the patient to look in the direction away from where the suture is located. For example, if you wish to remove a temporal corneal suture in the left eye, ask the patient to look to the right-hand side, as this will improve access and visibility of the suture.

- Approach the patient with the needle bevel facing away from the patient's eye.
- With the needle parallel to the corneal surface, slide it carefully between the suture and the ocular surface ensuring you do not damage the underlying tissue (Figure 10.4).
- Using the sharp edge of the needle, cut the suture on the opposite side to the buried knot, ensuring that your movement is away from the cornea.
- Now take the forceps and grasp the broken suture by the longest edge and pull the rest of the suture, including the knot, through the stroma and out (Figure 10.5). This ensures that the knot travels the shortest distance through the cornea possible and minimises the amount of suture being pulled through.
- If the suture breaks, then remove any exposed ends of the suture. Any unexposed suture in the corneal stroma can be left.

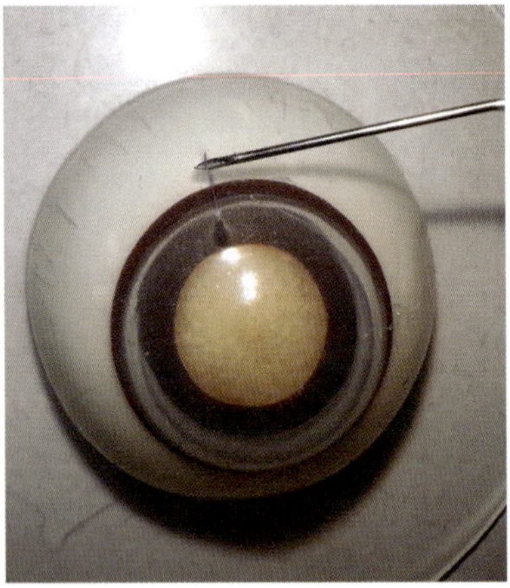

Fig. 10.4 Needle sliding between the suture and globe with bevel facing away from the patient.

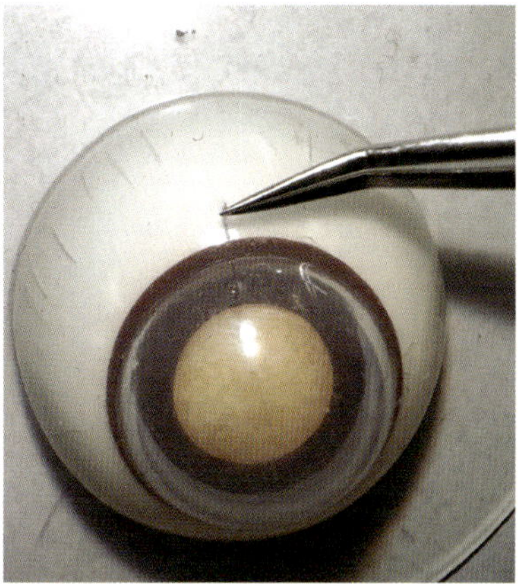

Fig. 10.5 Jewellers forceps grasping broken suture end.

POST-PROCEDURE

After removing the suture, apply a topical antibiotic such as chloramphenicol 0.5%. This can be given to the patient to use four times daily for a week to prevent any infection from developing. In cases of corneal graft sutures, topical steroids should be increased following the removal of sutures.

11

BOTULINUM TOXIN INJECTION

William Spackman

INTRODUCTION

Botulinum toxin is a neurotoxin produced by the *Clostridium botulinum* bacteria. It acts at the neuromuscular junction by inhibiting acetylcholine release and thereby paralyses muscle tissue. In ophthalmology, this action can be utilised to treat various conditions including blepharospasm, hemifacial spasm, entropion, aberrant regeneration of the facial nerve, strabismus and to induce a ptosis to protect the corneal surface.

Dysport and Botox are brands of botulinum toxin type A and are supplied in a dried formulation.[1] It is important to be aware of which botulinum toxin brand you are using as they have different reconstitution requirements and different dosage.

Botulinum toxin has peak effect at 2–6 weeks after injection and lasts up to 3 months. It is generally a safe and effective treatment and due to its temporary action, complications are unlikely to be permanent.

Specific injection sites and treatment regimens will vary according to which areas are affected and by clinician experience. Given the temporary action of botulinum toxin injection, patients with blepharospasm, for example, will require repeated injections at regular intervals. Therefore, a patient-specific treatment plan can be developed according to response to injections. Typically, injections are given into orbicularis at the "crow's feet" area and or brow but may also be given to the upper and lower lid depending on the patient's symptoms.[2]

In this chapter we hope to offer the basic principles of reconstituting Dysport and injection into the orbicularis muscle.

PRE-PROCEDURE

- A vial containing 500 units of Dysport is reconstituted with 2.5mL of sterile normal saline. This will give a concentration of 20 units per 0.1mL.[3]
  - Take a 5mL syringe and using a drawing up needle, draw 2.5mL of sterile normal saline.
  - Very slowly inject this into the vial of dried formulation Dysport, being careful not to inject too quickly or shake the vial as this may cause it to denature.
  - This vial should be kept refrigerated and used within 4 hours.
- Now take a 1mL syringe and draw up the required volume of reconstituted Dysport using a drawing up needle.
- In addition to the reconstituted Dysport, you will need:
  - Yellow 30-gauge needle
  - Sterile gloves
  - Gauze
- Ensure that the patient is comfortable, ideally on a reclined chair or couch with adequate lighting.

PROCEDURE

Injection into orbicularis:

- Securely place a yellow needle onto the 1mL syringe containing reconstituted Dysport.

- Identify the target area, place the skin on stretch and observe any obvious blood vessels in the area so that they can be avoided.
- Carefully advance the needle into the superficial, pre-tarsal orbicularis. When injecting into the brow, where the skin is thicker, the needle will need to be deeper to enter the orbicularis and pinching up the skin in this area may be helpful.
- Typically, 0.05–0.2mL is injected at each site but this can be adjusted and tailored over time according to response.
- Remove the needle and apply pressure to the area if there is any bleeding.
- Repeat the above in all required areas.

POST-PROCEDURE

Firstly, it is important to remind the patient that the response is not immediate. Typically, response may be seen from 1 day after injection, although this may take up to 2 weeks. Peak effect tends to be from 2 to 6 weeks and it can be effective up to 3 months.

It is important to assess how the patient responded to the treatment so that doses and injection sites can be changed. Over time, patients have been reported to develop antibodies to the botulinum toxin and so repeated injections may become less effective.

Potential Complications

The most common complication from botulinum toxin injections is bruising. This can be minimised with a good technique and by applying firm pressure at the site for 2 minutes if there are signs of bleeding.

Other complications include allergy, swelling, facial asymmetry, failure or incomplete response to treatment. Diplopia may occur if the extraocular muscles are affected, and ptosis is possible if levator palpebrae superioris is involved. Weakness of the orbicularis muscle may lead to poor eyelid closure, which has the potential to cause exposure keratopathy to the cornea.

Systemic side effects are rare but have been reported. Paralysis of muscles distant to the injection site is possible and this may therefore cause generalised weakness, dysarthria, dysphagia or respiratory failure if the diaphragm is affected. Since acetylcholine inhibition is the mechanism of action for botulinum toxin, the post-ganglionic parasympathetic nerves, some post-ganglionic sympathetic nerves, as well as the autonomic ganglia may be affected. This may cause side effects such as hypotension, urinary retention, constipation and reduced salivation, lacrimation and sweating.

Botulinum toxin should therefore not be given to patients with neuromuscular conditions such as Myasthenia gravis. It is also important to note that patients on aminoglycoside antibiotics such as Gentamicin will have an exaggerated response to botulinum toxin injections.

References

1. American Academy of Ophthalmology. Botulinum Toxin Use In Oculoplastics. Available at: https://eyewiki.aao.org/Botulinum_Toxin_Use_In_Oculoplastics [Accessed 20 Feb. 2023].
2. Bobs Korn (2021). 2021-2022 basic and clinical science course. Section 7, Oculofacial plastic and orbital surgery. San Francisco: American Academy Of Ophthalmology.
3. Dysport® (abobotulinumtoxinA) [Prescribing Information]. Cambridge, MA: Ipsen Biopharmaceuticals, Inc; July 2020.

12

LATERAL CANTHOTOMY AND CANTHOLYSIS

William Spackman

INTRODUCTION

Orbital compartment syndrome (OCS) or orbital apex syndrome is a true ophthalmic emergency and swift action in the form of lateral canthotomy and cantholysis can prevent permanent vision loss.[1] OCS can have a multitude of causes. It is most commonly seen in the context of blunt trauma resulting in retrobulbar haemorrhage and oedema. Patients at particular risk of OCS are those on anticoagulant medications or with clotting disorders. Other causes of OCS might include retrobulbar haemorrhage as a complication from peribulbar or retrobulbar anaesthesia and orbital cellulitis.

The eye is contained within the orbit, which is a fixed space. The orbital walls are made up by the orbital bones, which surround the eye in all directions apart from anteriorly, where the eyelids are positioned. This allows the eye some ability to protrude forwards in response to increasing mass within the orbit. Any increasing mass beyond this tolerance, will result in a rise in pressure within the orbit and cause ischaemic damage to the optic nerve.

In OCS, patients may describe eye pain, vision loss or double vision. However, some patients, particularly those who have sustained head trauma, may not be able to give a history and clinical signs are the key to diagnosis. These include proptosis, a sluggish or absent pupillary light reflex, a relative afferent pupillary defect, reduced colour vision, restricted ocular motility, periorbital bruising and subconjunctival haemorrhage.[2]

Orbital compartment syndrome is a clinical diagnosis and treatment should not be delayed to get radiological evidence. If there are signs of OCS, lateral canthotomy and cantholysis should be performed as soon as possible to prevent permanent visual dysfunction. Permanent damage may occur if the pressure is not released immediately.

If in doubt, it is always safest to perform a lateral canthotomy and cantholysis. It is a minimally invasive procedure with a low risk of complications and a serious risk of irreversible damage to the eye if not performed.

PRE-PROCEDURE

Ensure that all the required equipment is available before starting the procedure. You will need:

- Sterile gloves
- Local anaesthetic, e.g. lidocaine 1% with adrenaline
- Syringe and appropriate needle for drawing up and giving local anaesthetic
- Povidone-iodine or chlorhexidine
- Tenotomy scissors
- Forceps
- Artery forceps (mosquito)

If readily available, the following equipment may be helpful

- Diathermy
- Blade

Position the patient supine and ensure that there is space for you to access the head to perform the procedure.

PROCEDURE

Firstly, the anatomy of the area must be considered.

The lateral canthus is where the upper lid meets the lower lid, temporally. The lateral canthal tendon is attached to Whitnall's tubercle at the lateral orbital rim. As it travels medially, it separates into the superior and inferior crus. In a lateral canthotomy, the lateral canthal tendon is split horizontally. Cantholysis is then performed to cut the inferior crus. This should allow the lower lid to fall completely free of the eyeball and decompress the orbit. If this is insufficient, cantholysis of the superior crus can be performed.

Here is a guide to performing a lateral canthotomy and cantholysis:

- Firstly, administer topical anaesthetic to the ocular surface.
- Prepare the skin using povidone-iodine or chlorhexidine.
- Give subcutaneous local anaesthetic, ideally lidocaine 1% with adrenaline to help minimise bleeding. You will need to ensure that the areas at the lateral canthus and inferior to the lateral canthus are well anaesthetised.
- Crush the lateral canthus for 30 seconds using artery forceps (mosquito). This will minimise bleeding when a cut is made.
- Grasp with a pair of forceps just next to the lateral canthus and using a pair of tenotomy scissors in the other hand, cut through the lateral canthus and lateral canthal tendon. Extend all the way to the orbital rim (around 10–20 mm).
    - A blade may also be used to make a skin incision from the lateral canthus to the orbital rim, prior to cutting with the tenotomy scissors.
- If available, diathermy may be helpful to maintain haemostasis and help visualise anatomical structures.
- Pull the lower lid down using the forceps to reveal the inferior crus.
    - You can confirm the inferior crus by gently tapping it with a blunt instrument to feel the resistant, tendinous structure.
- Perform the inferior cantholysis by cutting through the inferior crus using the tenotomy scissors. Point the tip of the scissors away from the globe to reduce the risk of globe trauma.

- This should leave the lower lid completely mobile and may be sufficient to relieve the pressure within the orbit.
- If further decompression is required, a superior cantholysis can be performed by pulling the upper lid away and cutting through the superior crus. Care must be taken in a superior cantholysis to avoid the lacrimal gland.
- Apply a topical antibiotic ointment such as chloramphenicol 1% to the eye and wound.

POST-PROCEDURE

After completing the canthotomy, the eye should be re-assessed. If the orbit has been sufficiently decompressed within an appropriate time frame, you should hopefully see the vision improve, intraocular pressure reduce and the pupil become more reactive. If there is ongoing concern that the orbital pressure remains too high, further action may be required. This may involve giving intravenous acetazolamide or mannitol to lower intraocular pressure or further orbital decompression by a specialist.

The eye should be monitored frequently after the procedure, usually every 30 minutes for 4 hours initially, to ensure that the eye findings do not deteriorate again. Particular care should be taken in patients with clotting disorders or on anticoagulants as they are at particular risk of re-bleeding.

A topical antibiotic such as chloramphenicol ointment is usually given for at least a week following the procedure to reduce the risk of infection. The wound is usually self-healing, with minimal scarring and repair is not usually required but can be performed if necessary.

References

1. Bobs Korn (2021). 2021–2022 basic and clinical science course. Section 7, Oculofacial Plastic and Orbital Surgery. San Francisco: American Academy of Ophthalmology.
2. Hunt, S., Boulton, J. and Slade, T. (2019). Sight for Sore Eyes. [online] RCEM Learning. Available at: https://www.rcemlearning.co.uk/foamed/sight-for-sore-eyes/.

13

OCULAR SURFACE PROTECTION

Thomas Sherman

The ocular surface can become injured in many situations. Common examples include poor lid closure, e.g. due to Bell's palsy, corneal ulcers, surgical defects, chemical burns and many others. Here we describe some of the most commonly used methods of protecting the ocular surface, which can be applied across these different scenarios. They are used in combination with treatments directed at addressing the underlying pathology, e.g. antibiotics for infective corneal ulcers.

AMNIOTIC MEMBRANE

Amniotic membrane is an avascular foetal membrane derived from the placenta. Ordinarily, it is an immune-privileged site which prevents a maternal immune cell response reaching the foetus. Due to this immune privilege and natural avascularity, it provides a useful medium for a protective scaffold for the ocular surface. Fresh amniotic membrane from birth suites can be used; however, they are not permitted in the UK. Instead, freeze-dried amniotic membrane is used. Dried amniotic membrane can be obtained in forms such as Omnigen® (NuVision), which has the benefit of being able to be transported via post and then rehydrated.

Amniotic membrane has three important layers to its structure:

- Epithelial monolayer
- Inner extracellular matrix layer
- Chorion layer (this is the outer layer of the amniotic sac in utero)

Whether the epithelial layer is facing up or facing down alters how the amniotic membrane behaves when applied to the ocular surface.

Amniotic membrane can fulfill two functions (as shown in figure 13.1):

- **Patch:** Coats the ocular surface and cells proliferate under its cover. Provides a barrier to optimise healing environment. Epithelium side DOWN.
- **Graft:** Coats the ocular surface and becomes integrated into the tissue it is protecting as cells grow over the top. Replaces lost tissue. Epithelium side UP.

Two grafts may be combined with the epithelial sides in contact with each other to provide a combined graft and patch; cells will grow between the epithelial sides. Here there is the tissue integration function of a graft combined with the optimised healing environment that a patch provides. When using this technique, the overlying patch should have borders wider than the graft. Therefore, it may be necessary to remove some surrounding epithelium so epithelial growth does not become misdirected.

To work out which side is epithelium and which is connective tissue, the hydrated graft can have paper applied to one side. The non-epithelial side will produce a stringy material that sticks to the paper. The Omnigen membrane has a logo that orientates each side of the graft.

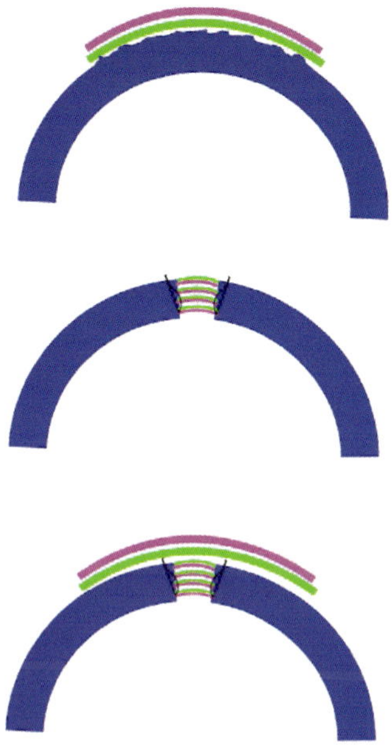

Fig. 13.1 The blue semicircles represent the cornea; pink is the non-epithelial side of the amniotic membrane and green the epithelial side. The top image shows a cornea with loss of the smooth epithelial surface; an epithelium-down patch has been applied to restore its integrity. The middle image shows the non-epithelial side down to create a graft that has been sutured either side of a corneal defect. A patch has been placed over this graft epithelium down in the lowest diagram.

Amniotic grafts/patches can be applied directly to the cornea or conjunctiva. There are different techniques to applying this outlined as follows.

Applying Amniotic Membrane

- **Suture** — 10-0 vicryl is usually used:
  For grafts this is placed partial thickness through cornea stroma after replenishing the lost stromal material with small pieces of amniotic membrane. Epithelium around the lesion should be debrided before applications.

Where a patch is placed, the amnion is laid over the corneal surface and sutured to the conjunctiva around 2 mm from the limbus. The patch usually dissolves naturally without need for removal.

- **Contact lens** — ProKera and OmniLenz are two examples of amniotic membrane integrated contact lens applications. For ProKera, the amnion comes integrated on a large-diameter contact lens, which is simply rinsed with saline and applied in the same way as a bandage contact lens. The OmniLenz system requires assembly with a provided contact lens and Omnigen disc. Both these systems can only be used as patches (i.e. epithelial side down).
- **Conformer** — Where a contact lens is not available, you can use a conformer wrapped in amnion. The hydrated amnion is first applied epithelium side down (as it is being used as a patch) and then wrapped around the conformer. An 8-0 vicryl suture is then used to secure the two sides of amnion together. Conformers are usually readily available in theatre so can be easily obtained.
- **Glue** — Cyanoacrylate or thrombin glue may be used. One technique described[1] involves cutting a 5 × 10 cm amniotic membrane sheet, trimming the upper and lower lid lashes, then gluing the membrane to the upper lid itself whilst using a symblepharon ring to achieve apposition of the membrane to the cornea. The lower half of the amnion is then stuck to the lower lid. Alternatively, glue can be directly applied to the cornea and the amniotic membrane placed on top (epithelium up as used as a graft).[2]

Applications

These are manifold, essentially wherever there is corneal layer loss or loss of conjunctiva, amniotic membrane can be considered. Some examples are detailed below:

- Cornea
  - Chemical injuries
  - Corneal ulceration (herpetic or bacterial) — Amniotic membrane may act as a sponge that concentrates the effect

of topical antibiotics where there is active infection, it also has anti-inflammatory effects that can benefit healing.[3]
  - Limbal stem cell deficiency
  - Bullous keratopathy
  - Stevens–Johnson syndrome
- Conjunctiva
  - Trabeculectomy bleb leaks
  - Exposed aqueous drainage device tubes (a double-layered amniotic graft/patch is used here)
  - Pterygium surgery
  - Chemical burns

FROST SUTURE

Frost sutures are most commonly used in maxillofacial surgery. Where cheek or lower lid skin grafts are created, the scarring process will eventually result in contraction of the lower lid itself, so a Frost suture is placed to counteract this downward traction. It was originally used to support the upper lid after ptosis surgery. There is variation in the exact way that Frost sutures are placed but it is usually a variation on the below:

1. Local anaesthetic is given to the lower lid.
2. 4-0 nylon (or similar non-dissolvable suture) is passed through the grey line or tarsus of the midpoint of the lower lid.
3. This can then be directly taped to the forehead. Alternatively, it can be fixed in place with a bolster.
4. The bolster is made from a small segment of venepuncture butterfly tubing. The suture is passed through forehead skin and then through the bolster and tied.

This provides lid closure. However, the force distributed in the lower lid is concentrated at one point. Therefore, there is a liability that the suture will erode through fairly quickly at this point. This may not be a major issue if only a few days of lid closure are needed. The other drawback is that instilling drops in a lid closed by a Frost suture is also difficult.

TARSORRHAPHY

There are several types of tarsorrhaphy, which can be subdivided into temporary and permanent. They can then be further subdivided into medial or lateral. Permanent tarsorrhaphies are performed in theatre by oculoplastic surgeons. It involves separating the anterior and posterior lamellae of the upper and lower lids, then fixing the posterior lamellae of the two lids together, before suturing the anterior lamellae together.

The temporary tarsorrhaphy is a useful technique that does not have to be performed in theatre. This uses a single suture to fix the upper and lower lids together laterally. However, a variable degree of lid closure is possible depending on how far along the lid the sutures enter and exit. The traditional method involves using bolsters and often describes placing sutures through the grey line of the lid. The grey line is made of weak muscle (muscle of Riolan) and does not provide as effective support as placing sutures through the tarsus. Bolsters can cause lash distortion and apply unwanted pressure around the lid margin, leading to necrosis. A much simpler, more efficient technique is described below:

1. Local anaesthetic is administered to the upper and lower lids.
2. Adson forceps are used to grasp the lid, and in doing so you will see meibomian secretions emerge, which guides you to the placement of the suture.
3. A double-ended 4-0 prolene suture is passed, one end passed through from the midpoint of the lower lid and emerging near the lateral canthus.
4. The other end is passed through the inverted upper lid (ensuring that the suture remains entirely within the tarsus) to emerge near the lateral canthus.
5. The needles can then be cut off and safely disposed of.
6. The two ends are tied (four throws are usually recommended to ensure no slippage) and the suture ends cut long

so that if there is migration of the suture material through the lid, there will not be a short barb injuring the cornea.

This technique was published by V. T. Thaller in an excellent article describing its use and the drawbacks of bolstered tarsorrhaphies.[4] The temporary tarsorrhaphy provides enough of an aperture to apply drops, whilst still protecting the ocular surface. Bear in mind that complete closure isn't always needed. Enough of a window can be left for a patient to see out of. Occasionally, if left in a long time, tissue may grow along the suture and form a thin column that remains when the suture is removed. This thin column of tissue can simply be cut and the lids will open normally.

BOTOX

This is fairly straightforward and involves injecting 15 units of Botox subcutaneously to produce a lowering of the levator palpebrae superioris. The needle is angled to be pointing along the length of the muscle as shown in figure 13.2 (i.e. pointing towards the patient as if injecting into the orbit, although orbital entry is not desired). The downside of this approach is that the ptosis can be variable in effect and duration. However,

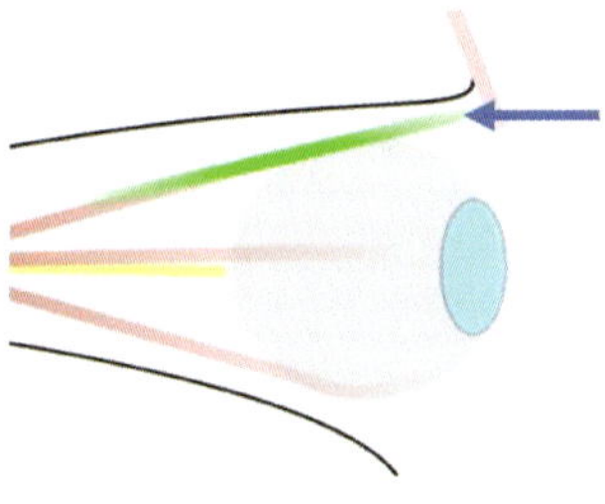

Fig. 13.2 The blue arrow shows the direction of travel towards the levator muscle shown in green. Aiming to go through the upper lid skin crease should allow you to reach the muscle, and deep penetration into the orbit is not needed.

it can be used in settings where the surgical methods of surface protection will not be tolerated.

CONCLUSION

There are multiple methods of achieving ocular surface protection, in all settings ensuring that adequate medical treatment (e.g. 2 hourly lubricant drops for exposure keratopathy and frequent topical antibiotic drops) is also required. However, these surgical techniques, if deployed at the right time, can promote a sight-saving healing environment for the eye to recover.

References

1. Shanbhag SS, Chodosh J, Saeed HN. (2019) Sutureless amniotic membrane transplantation with cyanoacrylate glue for acute Stevens–Johnson syndrome/toxic epidermal necrolysis. *Ocul Surf* **17**(3): 560–564.
2. Ahmad MSZ, Baba M, Pagano L, *et al.* (2022) Use of dried amniotic membrane with glue to manage a corneal perforation. *Eye* **36**(4): 894–895.
3. Ting DSJ, Henein C, Said DG, Dua HS. (2021) Amniotic membrane transplantation for infectious keratitis: a systematic review and meta-analysis. *Sci Rep* **11**(1): 13007.
4. Thaller VT, Vahdani K. (2016) Tarsal suture tarsorrhaphy: Quick, safe and effective corneal protection. *Orbit* **35**(6): 299–304.

SECTION II
LASER SKILLS

14

LASER FOR INTRAOCULAR PRESSURE CONTROL

Bryher Francis

There are two main laser treatments that can treat high intraocular pressure (IOP).

Firstly, a peripheral iridotomy in acute angle closure glaucoma (AACG). Secondly, routine selective laser trabeculoplasty (SLT) for long-term pressure treatment in chronic glaucoma. There are other laser treatments to treat IOP such as cyclodiode laser which are not covered in this chapter.

LASER PERIPHERAL IRIDOTOMY (LPI)

Introduction

In AACG, acute increased IOP is due to impaired outflow of aqueous humour secondary to appositional/synechiael closure of the trabecular meshwork, which leads to pupillary block. Although, we can treat the pressure with medical treatment, a peripheral iridotomy is the definitive treatment. It can break the current attack of AACG and prevent future attacks.

It is essential to perform this procedure as quickly after the diagnosis of acute angle closure is made, to prevent irreversible damage to the optic nerve. Gaining a good view for laser can be challenging, due to corneal oedema, flat anterior chamber and/or poor patient cooperation. Controlling the IOP medically will clear the cornea allowing laser to be performed safely.

It is always important to offer a LPI to the other eye. There is a 40–50% risk of developing AACG in the next 5–10 years.

Pre-Procedure

Explain the procedure to the patient. It is carried out under local anaesthetic and an iridotomy lens holds the eye open for the procedure. It takes around 5 minutes per eye. It should not be painful but patients describe an unusual "popping" sensation.

Consent should include: failure, further laser or surgery, bleeding causing blurred vision, inflammation, spike in eye pressure, glare.

Instill pilocarpine drops 30 minutes prior to the procedure to cause miosis and reduce the thickness of iris tissue. Warn the patient that these can cause headache. Instill an apraclonidine drop prior to treatment.

Procedure

Ensure that the machine is switched on and set up before the patient enters the laser room. Apply local anaesthetic drops. Peripheral iridotomy lens is required for the procedure with a coupling agent (Figure 14.1). The lens has an area of higher magnification, which allows you to see the area which you are treating in more detail. It also increases the power density by concentrating the laser energy. The lens also prevents blinking and minimises eye movement.

YAG (yttrium aluminium garnet) laser settings vary depending on the patient and their eye colour. Settings to start with 2–3 mJ, pulse 2. These can then be titrated accordingly.

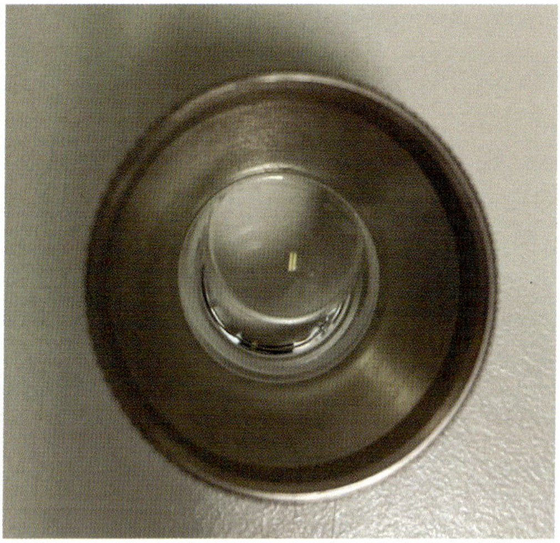

Fig. 14.1 Peripheral iridotomy contact lens.

The defocus should be set to zero. Aim for an iris crypt as this part of the iris is usually thinner, and therefore requires less power. Then offset the YAG beam so that it converges slightly posteriorly in the stroma.

Darker irises often require higher power as the iris tissue is thicker. Subsequent shots are administered to the same piece of tissue, until a patent hole has been formed. At this stage, you see a gush of aqueous humour with pigment into the anterior chamber. Avoid any obvious blood vessels as this will precipitate bleeding. Once the hole is patent, it can be widened slightly to reduce the risk of subsequent closure.

There are different trains of thought on the position of the LPI. Some clinicians perform LPI in superior quadrants between 11 and 1 o'clock (avoiding 12 o'clock as air bubbles in the anterior chamber can occlude this). It is thought that if it is located under the upper lid, then it should cause less glare for the patient. Other clinicians believe that superior LPI can get glare from the prismatic effect of tear film at the lid margin and therefore place LPI at 3 or 9 o'clock.

Post-Procedure

A further apraclonidine drop can be given if high powers were used. Check the IOP 45 minutes following the procedure.

Patients can be given topical steroids to reduce complications from post-operative inflammation (such as guttate dexamethasone 0.1% QDS for 2 weeks).

A further appointment should be arranged in around 6 weeks to assess the patency of the peripheral iridotomy.

SELECTIVE LASER TRABECULOPLASTY

Introduction

The aim of SLT is to increase aqueous outflow through the trabecular meshwork. However, the mechanism of this is not fully understood. It is thought that the energy produces an inflammatory cascade, which causes the trabecular meshwork to be rebuilt and function more effectively.

It is indicated in patients with open-angle glaucoma and tends to reduce IOP by around 30% when used as an initial treatment. It usually takes around 1–3 months.

Pre-Procedure

Explain the procedure to the patient. The aim of the treatment is to reduce IOP. Explain that around 80% have a good reduction in pressure. It tends to last for 2–4 years and the treatment can then be repeated at that stage.

Risks of the surgery include a spike in eye pressure, post-operative inflammation, hyphaema, worse vision from corneal or macular oedema.

Pre-operative apraclonidine is given.

Procedure

Ensure that the machine is switched on and set up before the patient enters the laser room. An SLT lens is required with a coupling agent (Figure 14.2).

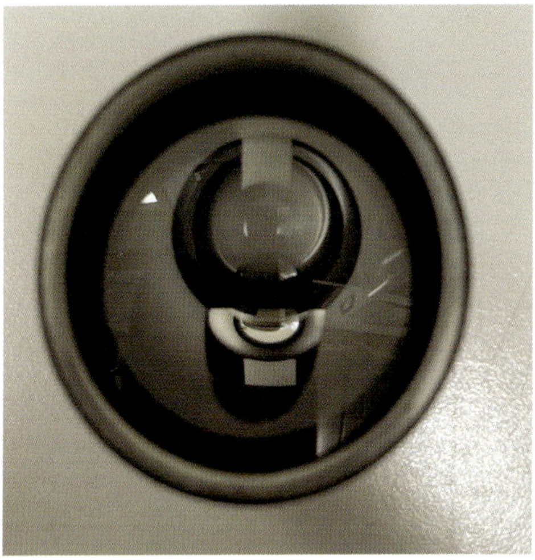

Fig. 14.2 Latina SLT lens.

The laser settings are fixed except for power. The aiming beam is centred over the trabecular meshwork. The aiming beam is out of focus when the surgeon is focused on the trabecular meshwork.

In lightly pigmented angles, the starting power can be set between 0.8 and 1.0 mJ. In heavily pigmented angles, the initial power can be lower at 0.4–0.6 mJ. The endpoint of treatment is the appearance of "champagne bubbles" adjacent to the trabecular meshwork. Ideally, these should be seen on every third shot. 360° of the trabecular meshwork can be treated in one session, normally with 100–120 shots per eye.

Post-Procedure

Post-operative apraclonidine is administered. Arrange for IOP to be checked 45 minutes following the procedure. Arrange for a follow-up appointment in around 6 weeks to monitor response of SLT.

15

LASER CAPSULOTOMY

Thomas Sherman

Laser capsulotomy is a common procedure in ophthalmic outpatients. It is usually performed to clear posterior capsule opacification (PCO) (Figure 15.1) from the visual axis to improve quality of vision. Here we will discuss how to perform a posterior capsulotomy safely. We will also touch upon some alternative capsulotomies performed.

POSTERIOR CAPSULOTOMY

Posterior capsulotomy is performed for PCO, which is a common problem occurring in around 5–20% of cataract cases after 5 years.[1] A YAG (yttrium aluminium garnet) laser with a 1064 nm wavelength is used for the procedure. Although sometimes posterior capsular opacities are cleared during vitrectomy, it is extremely rare for posterior capsular opacification to be treated this way, so there are no real alternatives to laser capsulotomy aside from not treating the PCO.

Consenting for Capsulotomy

The reason for capsulotomy is to improve vision. Formal risks that should be mentioned are inflammation, macular oedema,

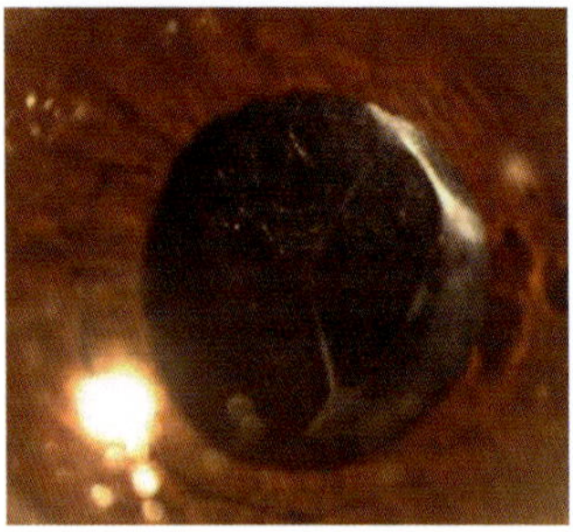

Fig. 15.1 Posterior capsular opacification of an intraocular lens (IOL). Note the string-like material on the anterior lens surface, which is a capsular remnant.

raised eye pressure, lens destabilisation, worse vision, retinal detachment. There are also some other key points to cover:

- The glasses prescription should not significantly alter.[2]
- The patient may experience an increase in floaters after the laser (usually decrease over a couple of weeks).
- The risk of retinal detachment is rare, estimated to be less than 1%.[3] Covering the non-intervention eye and checking there is no "curtain" type peripheral visual field disturbance is worth doing once a day for a couple of weeks post-laser.
- The laser is not painful but may be dazzling. Sometimes the vision is completely black and then comes back after a few minutes.

PERFORMING THE PROCEDURE

- Confirm the patient identity, laterality and procedure are correct compared to the consent form and medical record. Take particular care when you have a dual function machine that does both selective laser trabeculoplasty (SLT) and capsulotomy that the capsulotomy setting is selected.
- Apraclonidine/brimonidine pre- or post-procedure should be used.

Laser Settings

Offset: This refers to how far posterior to the aiming beam the laser has its focus. Some machines have pre-determined levels of offset and so the machine can only be set to "anterior, neutral, posterior". Set to posterior in these cases. Where a numeric offset is possible, usually this is set to between +125 and +250.
Power: As a general principle, the minimum amount of energy should be used. Sometimes if there is thin capsular opacity, a power as low as 0.3 mJ may be used. However, most of the time it tends to be between 0.5 and 1.0 mJ. It is rare to need to go higher than 1.3 mJ.

Technique

Once the patient's pupil has been adequately dilated with any dilating drop (tropicamide alone is usually fine), anaesthetic drops should be applied as well as topical apraclonidine 1% (iopidine). Before inviting the patient into the laser room, make sure the machine is all switched on and everything is working. It is not reassuring to patients if you are unsure about how to use the machine or equipment seems to be faulty.

Usually, a contact lens with artificial tear gel as a coupling agent is used, although it is possible to undertake a capsulotomy without a contact lens. Simply by increasing the magnification on the laser machine an adequate view can be achieved. However, most people probably do use a capsulotomy lens as it improves the view and avoids eyelids getting in the way.

The patient sits at the laser machine in the same way as a normal slit-lamp exam. Ensure that they are comfortable as the laser is difficult to perform with the patient moving around.

When ready to start the procedure, ensure that anyone in the room is wearing goggles of the appropriate filter and a light/sign alerting anyone outside the room not to enter is appropriately activated.

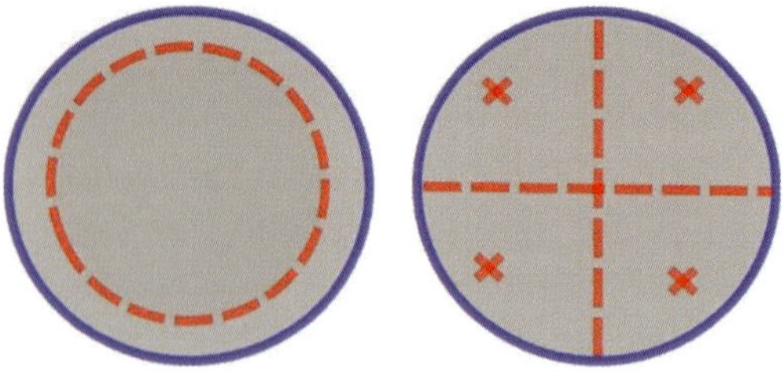

Fig. 15.2 Circle pattern on left and cruciate pattern on the right (with a few spots that usually need laser application to open central area further).

The aiming beam is adequately focussed on the posterior capsule, such that a single laser dot is seen, dragging the slit lamp back or forward to adjust the focus usually achieves this. For some laser machines I have found it to be easier to focus on certain areas with the patient looking to one side to obtain adequate focus. Patients have a tendency to close the fellow eye and this induces a Bell's phenomenon where the eye rolls upwards, so asking them to fix on a target or look down may be useful.

There are two main techniques to creating the capsulotomy (Figure 15.2). Creating a circle avoids any potential laser damage to the centre of the optic. However, it does create quite a large floater that may still require some central laser application to disperse. The cruciate pattern ensures that the central visual axis is adequately cleared (Figure 15.3) and leaves four leaflets to support the edges of the lens. However, this does mean applying laser to the central optical area. In addition to the cross pattern, a few shots usually need to be delivered to each of the four leaflets to move them out of the visual axis.

Aftercare

It is worth briefly inspecting to ensure that there are no straggling pieces of capsule floating around. If the patient has glaucoma, then an intraocular pressure (IOP) check after 30 minutes is advised. There is variation in the practice of prescribing post-operative steroid. In people with a history of uveitis, it is a good idea to give 4× a day dexamethasone 0.1%

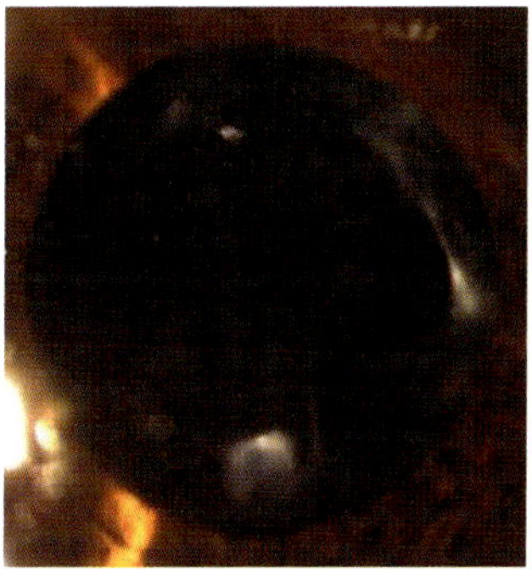

Fig. 15.3 Clear posterior lens capsule following laser.

or equivalent for 2 weeks, then twice a day for a couple of weeks. However, it is commonplace to not prescribe any post-operative drops in standard capsulotomy cases. If there are no other conditions needing follow-up, the patient can be discharged to their community optometrist after the procedure has been completed. Routine hospital-based follow-up after a capsulotomy is not usually needed.

Important Points

- Early posterior capsulotomy is best performed at 6 weeks postop or later to allow time for the eye to recover before having an additional procedure. An early capsulotomy is often required when polishing the posterior capsule has been difficult due to sticky soft lens material, which has remained stuck to the capsule at the end of cataract surgery.
- Beware of large IOP rises that can occur in glaucoma patients. It is best to check IOP 30 minutes post procedure for all patients with glaucoma.
- Take care where multifocal IOLs have been used as pitting of the lens can have significant refractive effects.
- Patients with a history of uveitis or cystoid macular oedema may have a flare up of these conditions after the procedure. Ideally, the laser should only be done when these conditions are quiescent.

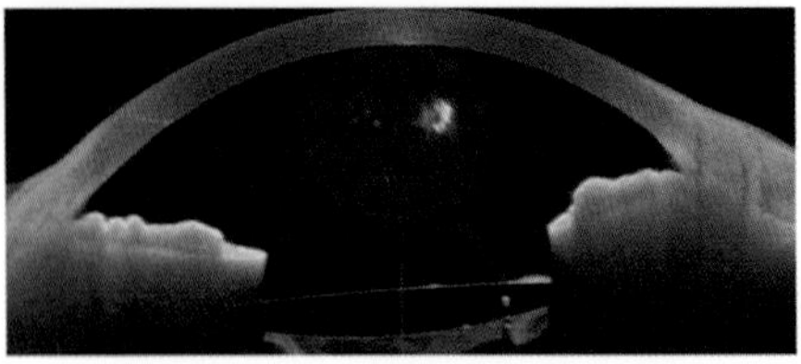

Fig. 15.4 A slit-lamp photo of a lens pit and corresponding location on anterior segment OCT.

Lens Pitting

One of the risks of YAG capsulotomy is the creation of lens pits. A photograph of one is shown in Figure 15.4 with a corresponding anterior segment optical coherence tomography (OCT) image. There is debate about the optical significance of these pits. Those not in the visual axis are highly unlikely to be visually significant. Even those in the central axis may not be noticeable to patients and are unlikely to cause problems.[4]

Capsular Block Syndrome

This condition can appear a few weeks after cataract surgery, or as a late-onset phenomenon. It is marked by the posterior capsule becoming dilated with turbid fluid. A posterior capsulotomy usually results in this dispersing and no long-term ill effect. However, patients may experience a change in refraction as the capsular distension induces myopia. In later onset cases, you may notice the capsular bag filled with bright white material. The temptation is to laser this with increasingly higher power, only to find very little progress is made. A good way of dealing with this thick material is to laser an area of clearer capsule to allow it to escape. You will see the white material get sucked back into the vitreous cavity and rise upwards as it is less dense than vitreous. Sometimes the material can completely obscure the view for further capsulotomy and you may need to plan a second laser another day. Topical steroids are best given in these cases as the material may be pro inflammatory. In addition, *Propionibacterium acnes* endophthalmitis can

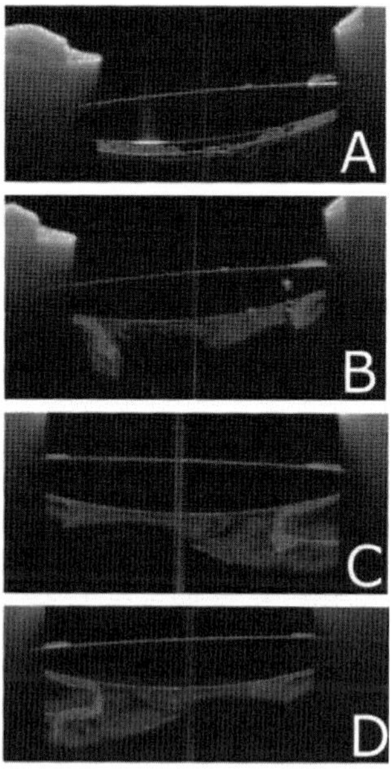

Fig. 15.5 Anterior segment OCT showing turbid material between the lens and posterior capsule (A). Immediately following laser (B–D) you can see how the capsule is reflected back on itself and this turbid material is floating around in vitreous. It will eventually disperse. When applying laser in such cases, any laser focussed onto the turbid material will simply move it around, and the posterior capsule needs to be broken to provide a means for it to escape.

present as a late-onset low-grade inflammation. There is often a white plaque on the posterior capsule, so consider this diagnosis if there are cells in the anterior chamber or vitreous. Figure 15.5 shows some mild accumulation of turbid capsular material, possibly retained soft lens matter, dispersing after laser capsulotomy.

ALTERNATIVE YAG CAPSULOTOMY PROCEDURES

Less common capsulotomy procedures include anterior capsulotomies and laser hyaloidotomy. Anterior capsulotomy is

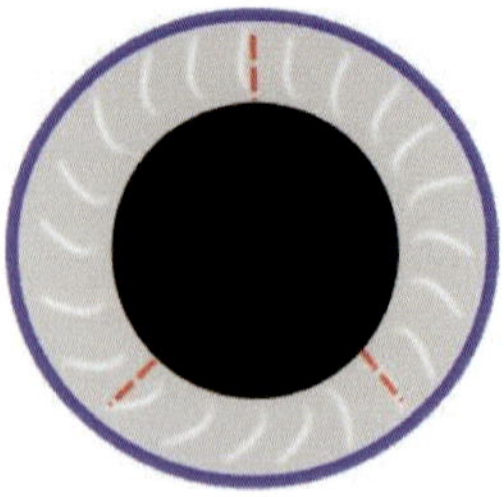

Fig. 15.6 Pattern for anterior capsulotomy (red dashes).

indicated in capsular phimosis. This occurs in cases where the surgical capsulotomy may have been created too small and can also occur in cases of retinal dystrophies which are associated with rapid proliferation of lens epithelial fibres.

In these cases, a hyperopic shift can result and so relieving tension on the capsular opening can correct this. Usually, a "Mercedes Benz" pattern (Figure 15.6) is made that breaks the capsular ring in three places. A laser power of around 1 mJ is typically needed with an anterior offset setting. A capsulotomy lens may be used. The endpoint of this procedure is when the fibrous ring has broken. Given that a fair amount of power and inflammation can be induced, it is important to give apraclonidine pre-procedure and 0.1% topical dexamethasone afterwards (usually 4× a day for a couple of weeks will suffice).

Laser hyaloidotomies are performed to disrupt the anterior hyaloid face in cases of aqueous misdirection. Usually, a laser power of 2–4 mJ is used to administer multiple shots (around 15),[5] aiming to disrupt the anterior hyaloid face which allows misdirected aqueous humour to drain freely. Consequently, the anterior chamber will deepen. Aqueous misdirection is a rare occurrence and it is advisable to get senior support in managing it.

CONCLUSIONS

Laser capsulotomies are relatively simple procedures to perform that can obtain great improvements in the patient's vision.

However, take caution in cases of glaucoma, uveitis and cystoid macular oedema as these can be aggravated. It is also a good idea to examine the fundus and potentially perform a macular OCT to rule out the possibility that problems other than PCO are causing reduced vision in cases where no pinhole improvement in acuity is seen.

References

1. Ursell PG, Dhariwal M, O'Boyle D, *et al.* (2020) 5 year incidence of YAG capsulotomy and PCO after cataract surgery with single-piece monofocal intraocular lenses: a real-world evidence study of 20,763 eyes. *Eye* **34**(5): 960–968.
2. Parajuli A, Joshi P, Subedi P, Pradhan C. (2019) Effect of Nd:YAG laser posterior capsulotomy on intraocular pressure, refraction, anterior chamber depth, and macular thickness. *Clin Ophthalmol* **13**: 945–952.
3. Wesolosky JD, Tennant M, Rudnisky CJ. (2017) Rate of retinal tear and detachment after neodymium:YAG capsulotomy. *J Cataract Refract Surg* **43**(7): 923–928.
4. Kruijt B, van den Berg TJTP. (2012) Optical scattering measurements of laser induced damage in the intraocular lens. *PLoS One* **7**(2): e31764.
5. Melamed S, Ashkenazi I, Blumenthal M. (1991) Nd-YAG laser hyaloidotomy for malignant glaucoma following one-piece 7 mm intraocular lens implantation. *Br J Ophthalmol* **75**(8): 501–503.

16

RETINAL LASER

William Spackman

INTRODUCTION

Thermal photocoagulation of the retina can be performed as a treatment for a number of conditions including retinal tears, diabetic retinopathy and vascular occlusions. LASER (light amplification by stimulated emission of radiation) is applied to the retina using an argon laser, diode laser or PASCAL (pattern scanning laser), which uses frequency-doubled Nd:YAG (neodymium-doped yttrium aluminum garnet). Laser energy is absorbed by melanin within the retinal pigment epithelium (RPE) and induces a burn to the retina. This causes tissue necrosis and creates a chorioretinal scar.

In pan-retinal photocoagulation (PRP) or sector laser, the aim is to ablate the areas of peripheral retina that are ischaemic because of conditions such as diabetic retinopathy and retinal vein occlusions. It is the ischaemic retina that is stimulating the production of vascular endothelial growth factor (VEGF), which is driving neovascularisation. Ablating these areas of retina reduces VEGF production and can lead to regression of neovascularisation.

Laser retinopexy is performed to reduce the risk of retinal detachment when there is a break to the retina. Creating a thermal burn and inducing chorioretinal scarring creates an adhesion between the retina and the underlying RPE. If this is done 360° around a break, retinal detachment can be prevented by stopping the progression of subretinal fluid.

Retinal laser can also be used at the macular in focal and grid photocoagulation. Laser energy can be applied either directly to leaking microaneurysms in focal laser or to an area of macular oedema in grid laser. The aim of focal laser to a microaneurysm is to ablate the leaking microaneurysm whilst grid laser is thought to stimulate pumping of subretinal fluid from the macula.

Retinal laser can be delivered via slit lamp, indirect ophthalmoscope or endolaser. In this chapter we will primarily focus on PRP and laser retinopexy delivered via slit lamp.

PAN-RETINAL PHOTOCOAGULATION

In PRP, the aim is to ablate the peripheral retina. The amount of laser applied may depend on the extent of disease and may be guided by fundus fluorescein angiogram (FFA).

Different clinicians will have different approaches to PRP, but in general, PRP should not extend beyond the superior and

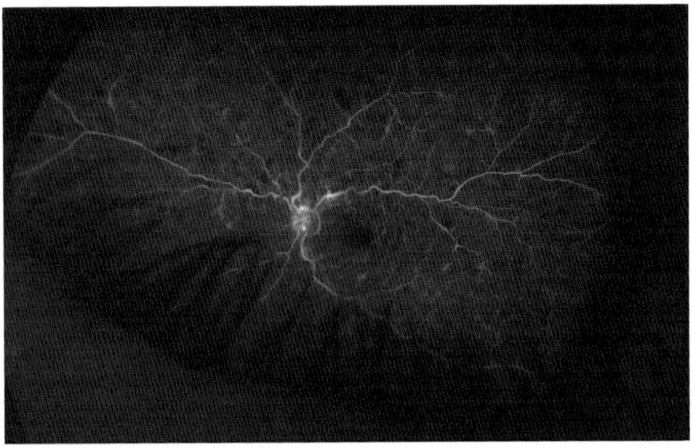

Fig. 16.1 FFA in a patient with a central retinal vein occlusion.

inferior temporal retinal arcades and not within 1 disc diameter of the optic disc nasally or within 3 disc diameters of the fovea temporally.

Pre-Procedure

Lens Selection

There are several different fundus contact lenses that can be used for PRP laser. Fundus contact lenses have the combined effect of stabilising the eye, keeping the eyelids open and focusing the laser on the retina with adequate magnification and field of view. Some of the more popular lenses for PRP include:

- Volk QuadrAspheric (120–144° field of view, 0.51× image magnification, 1.97× laser spot magnification)
- Volk Super Quad 160 (160–165° field of view, 0.50× image magnification, 2.00× laser spot magnification)
- Mainster PRP 165 (165–180° field of view, 0.51× image magnification, 1.96× laser spot magnification)
- Goldmann 3-mirror (140° field of view, 0.93× image magnification, 1.08× laser spot magnification)

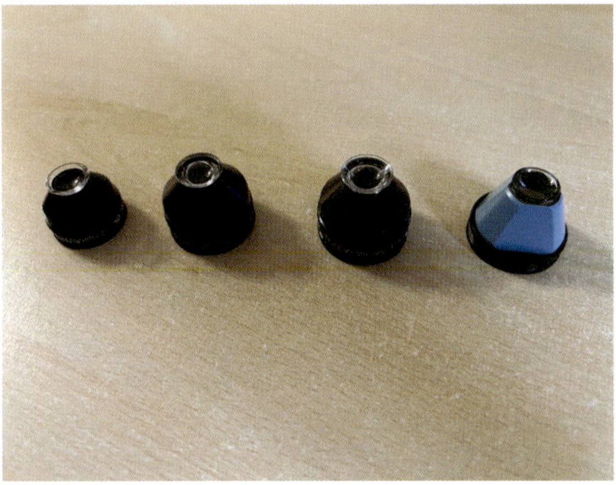

Fig. 16.2 Selection of PRP lenses; Volk QuadrAspheric, Volk Super Quad, Mainster PRP 165 and Goldmann 3-mirror (left to right).

Anaesthesia

In most cases, a topical anaesthetic is sufficient for patients to tolerate PRP laser. Oral analgesia such as paracetamol 1 g prior to the procedure may help. Some patients may experience more discomfort than others during PRP and completing it over several sessions may be necessary. In some cases, a periocular anaesthetic such as a sub-Tenon block is required. If this is insufficient, then indirect laser with sedation or a general anaesthetic may be required.

Laser Settings

Laser settings will vary between different machines, patients and areas of retina, and will need to be titrated according to response. Typically, with a PASCAL laser for example, a power of 250–450 mW, spot size of 200µm, and duration of 10–30 ms might be used. Senior advice should be sought locally to establish appropriate laser settings in your department. Various patterns can be selected to perform multiple shots with a single push of the foot pedal.

Equipment Required:

- Laser machine e.g. PASCAL laser
- Topical Mydriatics e.g. Tropicamide 1% and Phenylephrine 2.5%
- Topical Anaesthesia e.g. Proxymetacaine 0.5% or Oxybuprocaine 0.4%
- Fundus Contact lens
- Coupling gel e.g. Carbomer Gel

Laser safety rules and protocols should be followed at all times. Ensure all those in the room aside from the patient and yourself are wearing appropriate goggles, the laser warning light is activated and doors are locked.

Procedure

- Dilate the desired eye with mydriatic drops, e.g. tropicamide 1% and phenylephrine 2.5%.

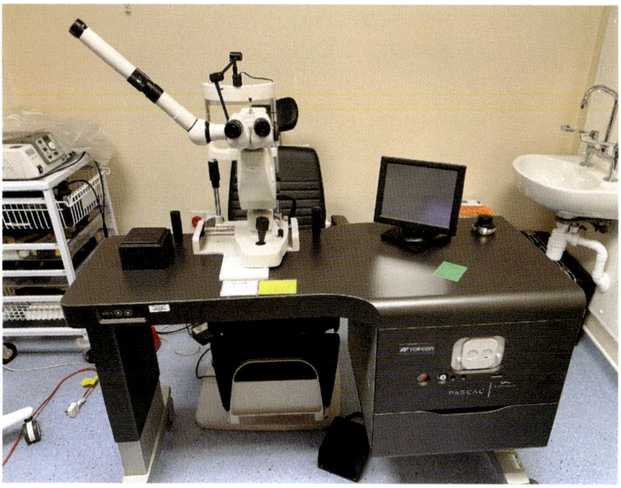

Fig. 16.3 PASCAL laser.

- Instil topical anaesthetic to the intended eye.
- Ensure that laser is on standby.
- Ensure that both yourself and the patient are comfortably positioned at the slit lamp with the patient's forehead firmly forward in the headrest.
- Place a small amount of coupling gel on the fundus contact lens ensuring that there are no bubbles and place on the patient's eye.
- Look down the slit lamp and take care to orientate yourself with the optic disc and macula.
  - It is imperative to know where these structures are at all times so that you do not accidentally laser the incorrect area of retina.
- Switch the laser to ready, which should activate the red guiding light.
- Starting with the peripheral, inferior retina, perform a test shot by pushing your foot on the foot pedal.
  - Start with a lower energy setting on single-shot mode.
  - You are looking for a light grey/white burn and should titrate the energy and/or duration up until an adequate response is seen.

  - Do not to use too much energy as this is more likely to lead to complications.
- When an adequate response is seen, and if the patient is tolerant and not prone to sudden movement, multiple-shot settings can be selected.
  - Shots should be at least one burn width apart.
- Laser the inferior retina first so that laser can be completed superiorly in the case of a vitreous haemorrhage developing.
- Then go on to complete the nasal, temporal and superior retina in turn ensuring that you remain:
  - At least 1 disc diameter away from the optic disc nasally.
  - At least 3 disc diameters away from the fovea temporally.
  - Not within the superior/inferior temporal retinal arcades.
- Patients are likely to be more uncomfortable when lasering the retina at the 3 and 9 o'clock positions as this is where the long ciliary nerves run.
  - Lower energy may be required or some clinicians advocate leaving these areas free. This may preserve some of the driving visual fields and reduce the risk of affecting pupil dilation and accommodation by damaging the long ciliary nerves.

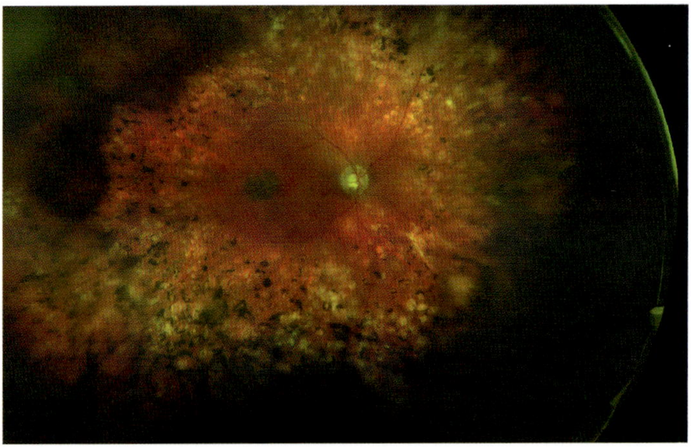

Fig. 16.4 Widefield fundus photograph of a patient with proliferative diabetic retinopathy who has had extensive PRP laser.

- There should be 2000–3000 laser burns to complete a PRP. This may need to be completed over several sessions.

Post-Procedure

Warn the patient that further oral analgesia may be required if there is discomfort following the procedure. Arrange follow-up to assess response to laser and arrange fill in laser if required.

LASER RETINOPEXY

In laser retinopexy, the aim is to surround a retinal break with burns to create a chorioretinal scar through which sub-retinal fluid cannot progress. Before performing retinopexy, you should thoroughly examine the retina to ensure that all retinal tears are identified.

Pre-Procedure

Lens Choice

The lenses detailed in the PRP section can all be used for laser retinopexy. Specific lens choice will depend on the location of

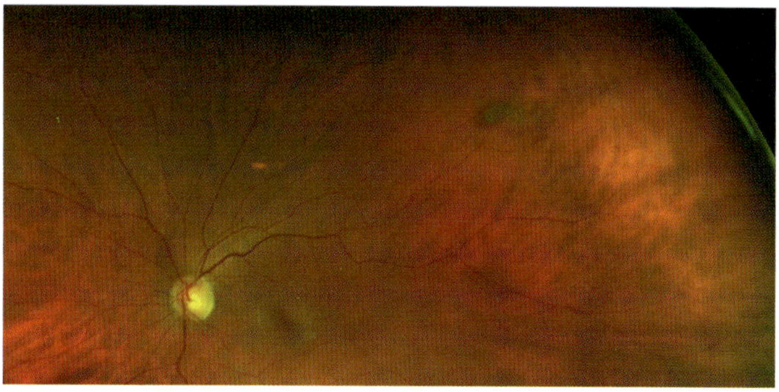

Fig. 16.5 Widefield fundus photograph of a patient with a superotemporal retinal break.

the tear and what field of view and magnification is required to visualise and adequately laser the tear.

Anaesthesia

Topical anaesthesia is usually sufficient to perform laser retinopexy but periocular or general anaesthesia may be necessary, particularly if scleral indentation is required with indirect delivery of the laser.

Laser Settings

As before, settings will vary and need to be tailored according to response. As a guide for the PASCAL laser, a spot size of 200μm, duration of 20-40ms and power of 250-450mW might be used. Senior advice should be sought locally to establish appropriate laser settings in your department. Single shot or multiple shot settings can be used.

Equipment Required:

- Laser machine e.g. PASCAL laser
- Topical Mydriatics e.g. Tropicamide 1% and Phenylephrine 2.5%
- Topical Anaesthesia e.g. Proxymetacaine 0.5% or Oxybuprocaine 0.4%
- Fundus Contact lens
- Coupling gel e.g. Carbomer Gel

Procedure

- Dilate desired eye with mydriatic drops, e.g. tropicamide 1% and phenylephrine 2.5%.
- Instil topical anaesthetic.
- Ensure that laser is on standby.
- Ensure that both yourself and the patient are comfortably positioned at the slit lamp with the patient's forehead firmly forward in the headrest.
- Place a small amount of coupling gel on the fundus contact lens and place on the patient's eye.

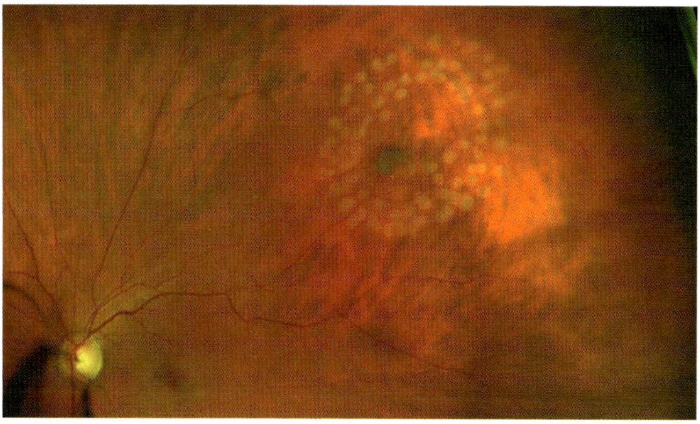

Fig. 16.6 Recently performed laser retinopexy surrounding the retinal break.

- Look down the slit lamp and take care to orientate yourself with the optic disc and macula.
- Identify the retinal tears to be lasered.
- Switch the laser to ready, which should activate the red guiding light.
- Perform a test shot around the tear and titrate the laser settings to produce a white burn.
- Proceed to place three rows of confluent laser burns 360° around the tear. Burns should be 0.5 burn width apart.
- In very peripheral tears, it may be difficult to get anterior to the tear and in these cases, indirect laser with scleral indentation may be required.

Post-Procedure

- Oral analgesia as required.
- Review in 1–2 weeks to ensure adequate uptake of the laser.
- It is important to note that the chorioretinal scars do not form immediately and there is therefore risk of progression of subretinal fluid in the early stages despite good laser. It is therefore important to issue a strong retinal detachment warning and advise the patient to present urgently should they get any new floaters, visual field defect or loss of vision.

COMPLICATIONS OF RETINAL LASER

It is important to counsel the patient on the risks and benefits of retinal laser prior to performing PRP or retinopexy. With PRP specifically, it is important to inform the patient that they will need to inform the DVLA and it may have implications on their ability to drive due to constriction of the visual field.

Great care should be taken to avoid inadvertently lasering an unintended part of the eye such as the cornea, iris, lens or fovea. Other complications may include corneal abrasion, oedema, vascular occlusions, vitreous haemorrhage and epiretinal membrane. Heavy burns are associated with progressive RPE atrophy, which is more significant, the more posterior the laser is applied.

References

1. McCannel C. (2021). 2020-2021 Basic And Clinical Science Course (BCSC): Retina and Vitreous Section 12. American Academy of Ophthalmology.
2. Sundaram V, Barsam, A, Barker, L. and Khaw, P.T. (2016). Oxford Specialty Training: Training in Ophthalmology. Oxford: Oxford University Press.

SECTION III
THEATRE SKILLS

17

BIOMETRY AND PRE-OPERATIVE CATARACT CONSIDERATIONS

Thomas Sherman

Understanding biometry is critical to a successful outcome in cataract surgery. Suboptimal refractive outcomes following cataract surgery can be a source of great disappointment and frustration to patients. Thankfully, modern biometry and lens power calculations are extremely accurate and limit the amount of "refractive surprise" that occurs post-op. Here we will explore how biometry is performed and the general approach to preparing for cataract surgery.

HOW IS BIOMETRY PERFORMED?

Most biometry is optical in nature, performed by non-contact techniques that measure axial length and keratometry as the two principal measurements of importance. These are used as part of formulae for calculating the power of intraocular lens (IOL) required to give a particular refractive outcome. The most widely used device is the IOLMaster 700® (Carl Zeiss). The IOLMaster 700® uses a swept source optical coherence

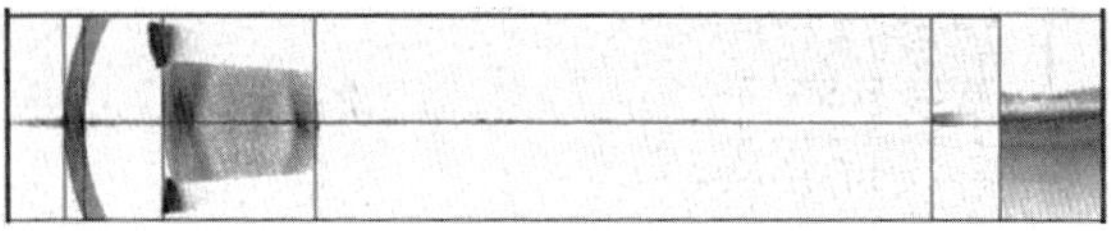

Fig. 17.1 OCT scan used to calculate biometry measurements for IOLMaster 700.

tomography (OCT) scan that measures from the corneal epithelium to the fovea. Therefore, as demonstrated in Figure 17.1, you can see exactly how the structures in the eye have contributed to the readout along the entire length of the scan.

Ensuring Accurate Biometry

Patients should keep soft contact lenses out for a week prior to having biometry. Hard contact lenses need to be removed for 2 weeks prior to measurement. Biometry is best acquired on a cornea that has had no ocular contact at that appointment, no tonometry or gonioscopy for example. If keratometry readings are difficult, sometimes a single drop of saline can improve the corneal surface. Artificial tears are more viscous and may distort keratometry readings.

Checking Biometry Results

1. Correct patient, correct eye, correct refractive outcome

Unfortunately, using the wrong biometry for the patient's cataract surgery still occurs. It is imperative to check three points of identification on all patients to ensure that you have the correct biometry for the right patient. Take time to work through in a stepwise way the name, date of birth, hospital number, date of biometry, eye to be operated on, refractive target and then think about what lens to choose. It is highly embarrassing for a patient to be on the table anaesthetised and only then to realise one of the identifiers is incorrect during the time out check.

2. Are axial length measurements accurate?

There should be six measurements taken for each eye. Missing values may mean that the biometry is inaccurate and should be repeated. Some people have a difference in axial length that exceeds 0.3 mm between each eye. Where this is the case, the machine will ask you to consider repeating the biometry. This is possibly a rather conservative estimate of the difference between the two eyes. However, it is worth checking where such a discrepancy is highlighted that the refraction matches this axial length difference (i.e. the longer eye is more myopic) this confirms that the measurements are expected.

3. Are keratometry measurements accurate?

A map is produced on the biometry report of the points used to produce the keratometry measurements, as shown in Figure 17.2. Where some of these points are missing or

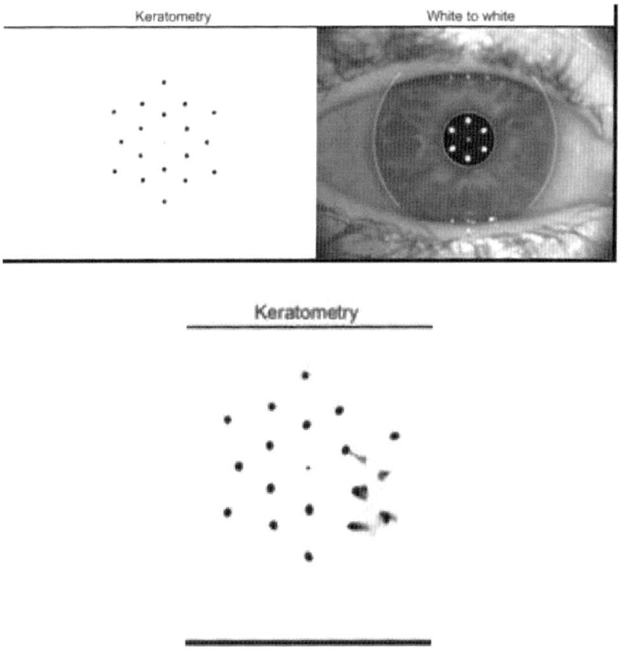

Fig. 17.2 Accurate keratometry depends on all LED points being crisp. the image on the left shows out of focus LED keratometry points that require repeating. The far-right image shows that a well-centred image with no interference in measurement from the eyelids was taken. The white-to-white measurement is the distance from the borders of the corneal limbus.

distorted, the quality of keratometry may be questionable. The green box below covers some of the important points regarding keratometry, which are also discussed in the corneal tomography chapter of this book.

Brief Overview: Keratometry

- Measurement of anterior corneal curvature*, taken from 18 reference points in approximately 1.5, 2.5 and 3.5 mm optical zones
- K1 is the flattest meridian
- K2 is the steepest meridian
- The degree of steepness is quantified with dioptres for each K value
- The axis of each meridian is stipulated in degrees (0° to 180° anticlockwise for each eye)
- The delta K is the difference between these values
- If operating "on axis", which is making the main incision for cataract surgery along the steepest meridian to reduce the amount of astigmatism, the axis of the K2 value is where the incision should be placed

**IOLMaster 700 now has a setting with "total keratometry (TK)" which combines anterior and posterior corneal curvature measurements with corneal thickness. Depending on what formulae your unit uses, they may use the standard K values or TK if using a formula like Barrett TK Universal II.*

4. Are the correct IOL selections available?

Other users of the biometry machine may have selected different lenses from the one you wish to use. Also note that the IOLMaster report can be either "multi formula" or "multi lens", so make sure the box you are selecting a lens from has the correct lens stipulated.

5. What formula should be selected?

Biometry formulas are the source of great research interest and much has been written about what formulas predict refractive outcome most reliably. The SRKT formula has been widely used for many years and remains so at the time of writing. However, there has been a shift to using Barrett Universal II formula in recent years in the UK. The Royal College of Ophthalmologists advises using formulas for the following axial lengths.

- AL $<$ 22.00 mm = Hoffer Q or Haigis
- AL 22–26.00 mm = SRKT or Barrett Universal II
- AL $>$ 26.00 mm = Haigis or SRKT

Remember that very long and very short eyes can also present surgical challenges. Long eyes often have deep anterior chambers that mean that the angle of approach to removing the cataract is more vertical. Short eyes can have smaller anterior chamber depths (below 2.5 mm is widely considered shallow), which restrict the space inside the eye to operate within and can result in more iris prolapse/posterior pressure. Refractive outcomes also become less predictable at extremes of axial length.

6. Selecting a lens

When you have decided which lens to use, mark it on the biometry sheet. Be aware that re-writing on a theatre list or whiteboard is an opportunity for transcription errors to occur. As such, it is best for the source document to be used if there are queries about what lens to use. In modern electronic notes systems, there is often a facility to select the lens electronically, which eliminates transcription errors. It is good practice to initial and date if you are hand selecting an IOL.

Summary of Biometry Checklist

Figure 17.3 shows the key areas to check before selecting a lens for a patient.

Navigating a Biometry Readout

We have covered the most important sections of the IOLMaster 700 report. However, it also contains other details that are rel-

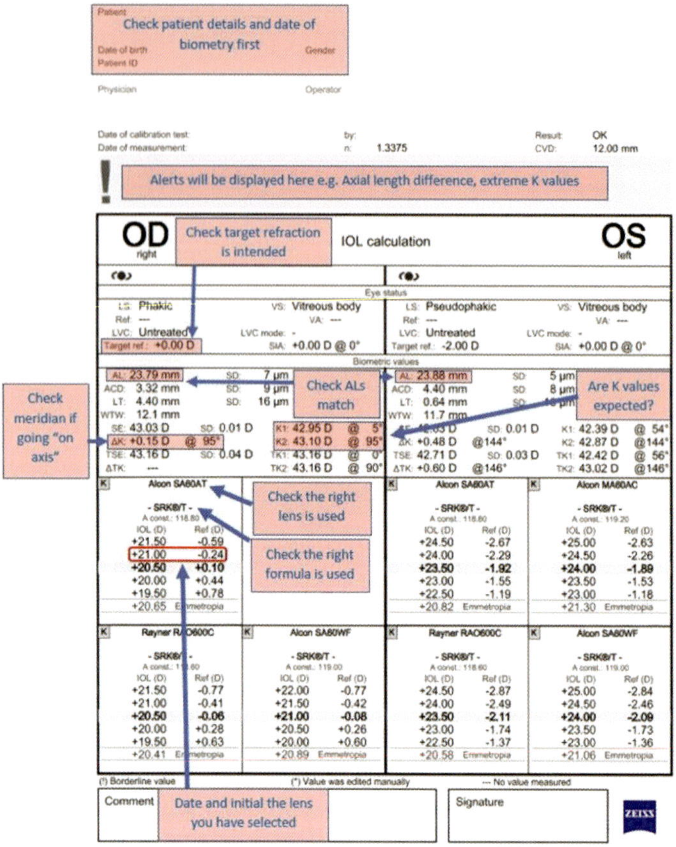

Fig. 17.3 IOLMaster 700 printout with important areas to check highlighted.

evant. There are usually several pages of information to each report:

- IOL calculation report (Figure 17.4): The main report for selecting the IOL.
- Individual eye analysis report (Figure 17.6): Contains details of the OCT and keratometry images to analyse.

Date of calibration test:	by:	Result: OK
Date of measurement:	n: 1.3375	CVD: 12.00 mm

! OD: Keratometry value is uncertain.

OD right — IOL calculation — **OS** left

Eye status

OD		OS	
LS: Phakic	VS: Vitreous body	LS: Phakic	VS: Vitreous body
Ref: ---	VA: ---	Ref: ---	VA: ---
LVC: Untreated	LVC mode: -	LVC: Untreated	LVC mode: -
Target ref.: +0.00 D	SIA: +0.00 D @ 0°	Target ref.: +0.00 D	SIA: +0.00 D @ 0°

Biometric values

OD				OS			
AL: 23.90 mm	SD: 7 µm			AL: 23.81 mm	SD: 8 µm		
ACD: 3.23 mm	SD: 6 µm			ACD: 3.25 mm	SD: 6 µm		
LT: 4.63 mm	SD: 13 µm			LT: 4.66 mm	SD: 41 µm		
WTW: 12.1 mm				WTW: 12.1 mm (!)			
SE: 42.23 D	(!) SD: 0.02 D	K1: 42.04 D	@119°	SE: 42.81 D	SD: 0.01 D	K1: 42.48 D	@ 31°
ΔK: +0.38 D	@ 29°	K2: 42.42 D	@ 29°	ΔK: +0.66 D	@121°	K2: 43.14 D	@121°
TSE: 42.23 D	(!) SD: 0.05 D	TK1: 41.95 D	@107°	TSE: 42.85 D	SD: 0.03 D	TK1: 42.48 D	@ 42°
ΔTK: +0.56 D	@ 17°	TK2: 42.51 D	@ 17°	ΔTK: +0.75 D	@132°	TK2: 43.23 D	@132°

OD: Alcon SA60AT		OD: Alcon MA60AC		OS: Alcon SA60AT		OS: Alcon MA60AC	
- SRK®/T -		- SRK®/T -		- SRK®/T -		- SRK®/T -	
A const.: 118.80		A const.: 119.20		A const.: 118.80		A const.: 119.20	
IOL (D)	Ref (D)	IOL (D)	Ref (D)	IOL (D)	Ref (D)	IOL (D)	Ref (D)
+22.00	-0.57	+22.50	-0.57	+22.00	-0.82	+22.50	-0.82
+21.50	-0.22	+22.00	-0.22	+21.50	-0.47	+22.00	-0.47
+21.00	**+0.13**	**+21.50**	**+0.12**	**+21.00**	**-0.12**	**+21.50**	**-0.13**
+20.50	+0.48	+21.00	+0.46	+20.50	+0.22	+21.00	+0.21
+20.00	+0.82	+20.50	+0.80	+20.00	+0.56	+20.50	+0.54
+21.19	Emmetropia	+21.68	Emmetropia	+20.82	Emmetropia	+21.31	Emmetropia

OD: Alcon A/C Lens		OD: Alcon SA60WF		OS: Alcon A/C Lens		OS: Alcon SA60WF	
- SRK®/T -		- SRK®/T -		- SRK®/T -		- SRK®/T -	
A const.: 115.20		A const.: 119.00		A const.: 115.20		A const.: 119.00	
IOL (D)	Ref (D)	IOL (D)	Ref (D)	IOL (D)	Ref (D)	IOL (D)	Ref (D)
+18.50	-0.86	+22.50	-0.75	+18.00	-0.72	+22.00	-0.65
+18.00	-0.45	+22.00	-0.40	+17.50	-0.31	+21.50	-0.30
+17.50	**-0.03**	**+21.50**	**-0.05**	**+17.00**	**+0.10**	**+21.00**	**+0.04**
+17.00	+0.38	+21.00	+0.30	+16.50	+0.50	+20.50	+0.38
+16.50	+0.78	+20.50	+0.64	+16.00	+0.90	+20.00	+0.72
+17.46	Emmetropia	+21.43	Emmetropia	+17.12	Emmetropia	+21.07	Emmetropia

(!) Borderline value (*) Value was edited manually --- No value measured

Comment

Signature

ZEISS

IOLMaster 700 Version 1.90.12.05 Report dated Page 1 of 6

Fig. 17.4 IOL calculation report.

AL: 23.90 mm	SD: 7 µm				
ACD: 3.23 mm	SD: 6 µm				
LT: 4.63 mm	SD: 13 µm				
WTW: 12.1 mm					
SE: 42.23 D	(!) SD: 0.02 D	K1: 42.04 D	@119°		
ΔK: +0.38 D	@ 29°	K2: 42.42 D	@ 29°		
TSE: 42.23 D	(!) SD: 0.05 D	TK1: 41.95 D	@107°		
ΔTK: +0.56 D	@ 17°	TK2: 42.51 D	@ 17°		

Fig. 17.5 Biometric values.

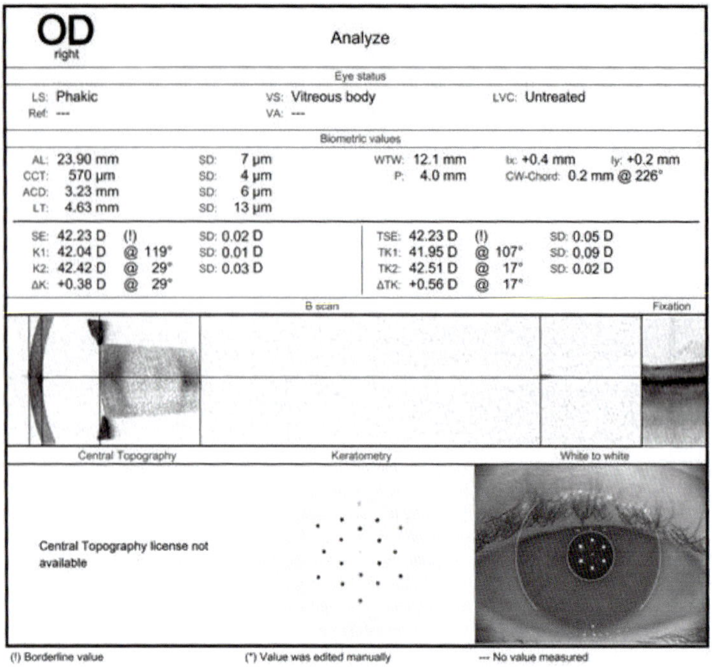

Fig. 17.6 Individual eye analysis report.

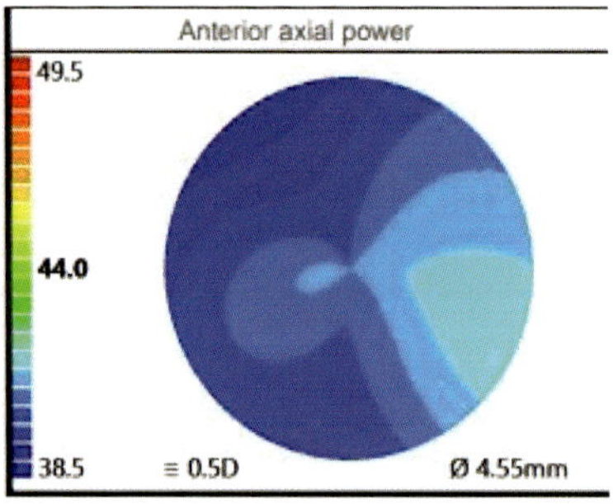

Fig. 17.7 Corneal topography reading showing an overall rather flat cornea in all meridians.

- Steep meridian map (Figure 17.8): Same data as individual eye analysis but with a map projecting the orientation of the steep axis.
- Summary of all biometric values (Figure 17.9): Contains all individual measurements taken so that every individual

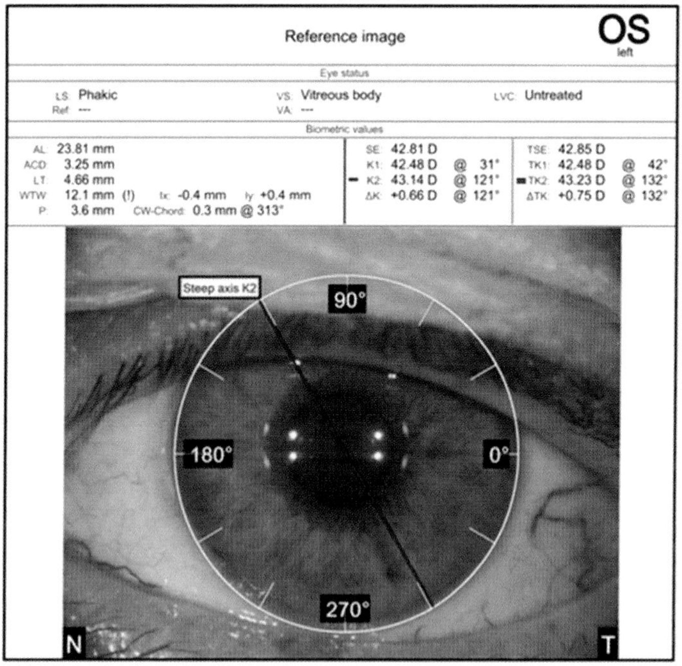

Fig. 17.8 Map of steep meridian to guide incision placement. Some operating microscopes have a facility to project this onto the eye during surgery.

reading can be interrogated. For example, to arrive at the final axial length measurement, three readings are taken in six meridians, and these data are available on the summary sheet.

IOL Calculation Report

In the following subsection we will run through the parameters on the printout not covered in Figure 17.3. These parameters often are areas used by specialists or represent fields that are not usually changed. However, it is useful to have some understanding of what they mean.

- N this is the cornea's refractive index used for calculating K values.

OD right	Biometric values	**OS** left

Eye status

OD		OS	
LS: Phakic	VS: Vitreous body	LS: Phakic	VS: Vitreous body
Ref: ---	VA: ---	Ref: ---	VA: ---
LVC: Untreated		LVC: Untreated	

Biometric values

OD		OS	
AL: **23.90** mm	SD: 7 µm	AL: **23.81** mm	SD: 8 µm
CCT: **570** µm	SD: 4 µm	CCT: **596** µm	SD: 5 µm
ACD: **3.23** mm	SD: 6 µm	ACD: **3.25** mm	SD: 6 µm
LT: **4.63** mm	SD: 13 µm	LT: **4.66** mm	SD: 41 µm

AL	CCT	ACD	LT	AL	CCT	ACD	LT
23.89 mm	571 µm	3.23 mm	4.63 mm	23.82 mm	597 µm	3.25 mm	4.60 mm
23.90 mm	565 µm	3.22 mm	4.64 mm	23.81 mm	593 µm	3.25 mm	4.67 mm
23.90 mm	570 µm	3.22 mm	4.62 mm	23.81 mm	594 µm	3.26 mm	4.66 mm
23.90 mm	573 µm	3.23 mm	4.63 mm	23.81 mm	593 µm	3.25 mm	4.68 mm
23.90 mm	571 µm	3.23 mm	4.64 mm	23.82 mm	603 µm	3.25 mm	4.68 mm
23.89 mm	571 µm	3.23 mm	4.62 mm	23.81 mm	598 µm	3.25 mm	4.66 mm

Corneal values

OD			OS		
SE: **42.23** D	(!)	SD: 0.02 D	SE: **42.81** D		SD: 0.01 D
K1: **42.04** D	@ **119°**	SD: 0.01 D	K1: **42.48** D	@ **31°**	SD: 0.01 D
K2: **42.42** D	@ **29°**	SD: 0.03 D	K2: **43.14** D	@ **121°**	SD: 0.03 D
ΔK: **+0.38** D	@ **29°**		ΔK: **+0.66** D	@ **121°**	
SE: 42.24 D	ΔK: +0.39 D	@ 30°	SE: 42.80 D	ΔK: +0.64 D	@ 121°
SE: 42.24 D	ΔK: +0.40 D	@ 29°	SE: 42.81 D	ΔK: +0.64 D	@ 121°
SE: 42.21 D	ΔK: +0.36 D	@ 30°	SE: 42.82 D	ΔK: +0.69 D	@ 121°
TSE: **42.23** D	(!)	SD: 0.05 D	TSE: **42.85** D		SD: 0.03 D
TK1: **41.95** D	@ **107°**	SD: 0.09 D	TK1: **42.48** D	@ **42°**	SD: 0.05 D
TK2: **42.51** D	@ **17°**	SD: 0.02 D	TK2: **43.23** D	@ **132°**	SD: 0.10 D
ΔTK: **+0.56** D	@ **17°**		ΔTK: **+0.75** D	@ **132°**	
TSE: 42.27 D	ΔTK: +0.53 D	@ 17°	TSE: 42.82 D	ΔTK: +0.66 D	@ 133°
TSE: 42.26 D	ΔTK: +0.51 D	@ 22°	TSE: 42.86 D	ΔTK: +0.66 D	@ 133°
TSE: 42.17 D	ΔTK: +0.64 D	@ 14°	TSE: 42.88 D	ΔTK: +0.91 D	@ 132°

White-to-white and pupil values

OD		OS	
WTW: 12.1 mm	Ix: +0.4 mm Iy: +0.2 mm	WTW: 12.1 mm (!)	Ix: -0.4 mm Iy: +0.4 mm
P: 4.0 mm	CW-Chord: 0.2 mm @ 226°	P: 3.6 mm	CW-Chord: 0.3 mm @ 313°

Image stored (!)	Reference image	Image stored

Fig. 17.9 Biometry summary. A (!) symbol means there is a borderline value with a lower signal:noise ratio that should be checked for plausibility with the other values. It does not necessarily mean that the reading is incorrect.

- The CVD is the corneal vertex distance which is used in OCT machine biometry calculations.
- LS: Lens status.
- LVC: If there has been a history of laser refractive surgery (laser vision correction), it can be entered here. The IOLMaster allows a choice of LASIK, LASEK, PRK and an LVC mode of hyperopic or myopic. The Haigis L formula will then be selected by the machine. Please note that patients with previous refractive surgery are not straightforward cataract cases and it is best to speak with your supervisor about the best management for these patients.
- SIA: Surgically induced astigmatism: if the surgeon knows how much astigmatism is induced through their technique,

they can enter it manually into the IOLMaster and it will be used in determining the optimum lens choice. As most NHS practices have multiple users, this is generally left at 0.
- VA and Ref: Visual acuity and refraction can be entered onto the IOLMaster, this is seldom done.

The biometric values (Figure 17.5) include some additional measurements we have not previously mentioned. The lens thickness (LT) is the distance from the anterior to posterior poles of the lens. LT is used in fourth generation formulae (e.g. Haigis, Holladay 2) to work out the effective lens position. ELP is important as it is the ultimate position the lens will end up following surgery. SRKT and similar generation formulae work out ELP by using axial length and keratometry values. However, the inclusion of more parameters can improve ELP prediction. Improving precision of ELP prediction is an area of ongoing research, but it is useful to be familiar with the concept of ELP as you will encounter patients who initially have “perfect vision” only to then find that they require glasses to see clearly, despite no post-operative pathology. This is usually due to a shift in ELP as the capsule has contracted post-surgery.

White-to-white values are used to plan anterior chamber lens insertion. Generally, one adds 1 mm onto the white-to-white distance to find the appropriate length anterior chamber IOL. The keratometry values on the IOL printout have previously been discussed. Note that if this reading states “keratometry value is uncertain”, it doesn’t necessarily mean the reading is incorrect, but rather should be checked for plausibility. This can result if the readings from the optical zones do not appear to show consistency.

You can compare K readings to a corneal tomography (e.g. Pentacam readout). However, the two are not directly comparable. Although K values can be entered manually from tomography data, there are proprietary manipulations of the IOLMaster K readings that are used to generate total cornea refractive power. These calculations are not possible with manually entered data, so any data inputted in this way will flag an alert on the printout.

Individual Eye Analysis Report

Many of these parameters have already been discussed. However, there are some that are unique to this report:

- CW-Chord (Chang–Waring) — This is a measurement of angle kappa, the difference between the visual axis (a line from object to fovea) and the pupil axis (a line through the centre of the pupil). This angle can have implications for the centration of premium lenses (mainly multifocal or extended-depth-of-field IOL's with diffractive rings). Whilst this is an ongoing area of study, it is thought that a value above 0.6 mm is more likely to lead to post-operative haloes and glare with such IOL's. For monofocal lenses used on the NHS, this is not really a concern. Two values for the corneal apex and centration are then provided for similar reasons relating to centration.
- Lx — Shift of corneal apex towards iris centre in X axis
- Ly — Shift of corneal apex towards iris centre in Y axis
- P — Pupil diameter in millimeter
- CCT — Central corneal thickness

Additionally, the IOLMaster 700 now has a corneal topography licence to display the central corneal topography. When enabled, a map such as that shown in Figure 17.7 will display. The corneal tomography chapter discusses more about how to interpret such heat maps.

The remaining two IOLMaster 700 printouts do not contain any additional measurements not already discussed, but are included here for completeness.

MANUAL BIOMETRY

This uses A scan ultrasound to measure the axial length and a handheld keratometer (or K readings from the IOLMaster) to calculate the lens required. Often the A scan machines are purpose built for biometry use. They usually have software built into them to calculate a selection of lens powers to achieve a given refraction. The technicalities of A scan biometry are discussed in the ultrasound chapter of this book. Manual biometry may be done on the operating table in children or patients with advanced dementia/learning difficulties who are not able to tolerate optical biometry. However, you need to be mindful that a great deal more operator-dependant variables can be introduced as sources of error here.

CONSIDERATIONS WHEN LISTING PATIENTS FOR CATARACT SURGERY

Following on from biometry interpretation, it is important when doing a cataract clinic to think about how to optimise the chances of a patient achieving a good result from surgery and being satisfied with their post-op visual outcome.

Specific Points to Cover

The following is a list of particular points to think about when listing someone for cataract surgery that should hopefully maximise the chances of achieving a good outcome for the patient.

Is this patient symptomatic of cataract?

Unless cataract surgery is needed for intraocular pressure control or narrow-angle glaucoma, cataract surgery should only be done for patients having day-to-day problems with their sight.

Have you discussed the refractive outcome?

This is absolutely imperative to do. Sadly, you will still come across instances where it is not done. If you notice this to be the case in advance of surgery, call the patient and discuss refractive outcomes with them. If in your clinic you do not have time to discuss this, schedule a telephone consultation to discuss it at a later date. Consider restructuring your cataract counselling to prioritise discussing this next time. Time and again refractive dissatisfaction occurs post-cataract surgery.

This may be an unavoidable "refractive surprise". However, there are undoubtably instances where inadequate discussions about spectacle dependence post-operatively have resulted in disappointed patients whose expectations have not been understood. Different patients need different discussions.

Low Hyperopia/Low Myopia (+1 to –1)

Most patients will have an emmetropic target. They need to be aware that reading glasses will be needed following surgery.

Moderate/High Hyperopia

Hyperopes will usually benefit from having their hyperopia removed. However, you need to warn them about potential anisometropia post-op which can cause a "sea sick" feeling of imbalance. Generally, patients at risk of this are ones who will have 2 dioptres of difference between the two eyes. However, individual tolerances may vary.

Moderate Myopia (–2 to –4)

These patients often take their glasses off to read. Most want to keep this ability (around –2 is suitable for this purpose. However, some may target slightly less myopia than this). Some want to have better vision for distance. Around –1 is a good level of myopia that will mean a need to wear driving glasses but reasonable intermediate vision/distance vision. Beware aiming for less than –0.5 dioptres as converting a myope to hyperopia will make them very unhappy.

These patients may also be suitable for monovision (setting one eye for near and one for distance). However, this is not for everyone and best practice is to have a contact lens trial of this to see if the difference between the two eyes is tolerated. However, cataract may fog the vision and impede the accuracy of this trial. If the patient has a "dominant" eye, this generally should be set for emmetropia and the fellow eye may then be set for a near target if monovision is desired.

High Myopia (–5 and Beyond)

Many high myopes wear contact lenses and may be keen to get rid of these. They may be so myopic that they keep glasses on for reading and depending on their work/hobbies may want to have good distance vision. You need some idea of whether the patient would prefer to aim to be glasses free for near or distance. With very high levels of myopia, e.g. −10, refractive outcomes start to become less certain and it is important to emphasise that glasses may well be needed for distance and reading post-op. It is probably unwise to aim for anything closer to 0 than −1 if the patient is after good "distance vision". Oftentimes, the fellow eye is also very myopic and may need surgery to balance the two eyes.

NB: These are not cast iron rules and different surgeons will have different targets they will aim for with myopes. If in doubt about refractive target, discuss. It is far better to have a discussion than to learn from mistakes of "having a go" and compromising patient's quality of life in the process.

Astigmatic patients will need to be warned that they may require distance and reading glasses unless there is a plan to insert a toric lens.

A history of refractive surgery is important to specifically ask about. Refractive surgery alters the relationship between the anterior and posterior corneal curvature and will require lens calculation using a purpose-made calculator. A commonly used one is available for free from the American Society of Cataract and Refractive Surgery (https://iolcalc.ascrs.org/). Refractive outcomes can be unpredictable in these patients, and given they have paid to be spectacle free in the past, they need to be warned that spectacles may be necessary following cataract surgery.

Have you elicited risk factors particular to the patient that may make surgery difficult?

These include the use of alpha blockers like tamsulosin or doxazosin that can result in floppy iris, poorly dilating pupils, loose zonules (the lens can be seen to wobble inside the eye if

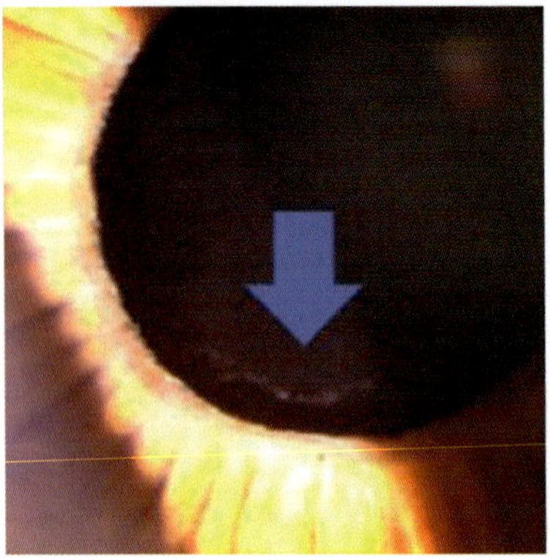

Fig. 17.10 Pseudoexfoliation on an IOL surface. Note the subtle material on the pupil rim, this is important to actively look for as it is easily missed and is associated with weak zonules.

the patient looks around, termed phacodonesis) and an inability to lie flat. Figure 17.10 shows pseudoexfoliation which indicates cataract surgery may be complicated by lens instability.

Have you discussed the material risks and benefits to the patient?

The usual quoted risks are:

- 1:1000 risk of blindness from infection, bleeding or retinal detachment
- 1:100 (variable) of need for further surgery due to complications during surgery, e.g. posterior capsular rupture
- 1:20 risk of post-operative inflammation, cystoid macular oedema or other problem delaying postop recovery
- 1:10 risk of needing laser in the future for posterior capsular opacification
- Risk of needing distance as well as reading glasses (depends on individual patient)

Less frequently discussed risks that are still relevant to patients include: risk of exacerbation of dry eye, risk of negative dysphotopsia (a dark crescent in temporal visual field from the edge of the IOL), lid position abnormalities induced by the speculum (e.g. ptosis or ectropion) and alteration of colour perception (blue objects appear more blue, which can be relevant to artists/painters).

Have you discussed choice of anaesthetic?

The vast majority of patients are suitable for local anaesthesia. It is important to make them aware that they are awake, but will only be able to see shadows/colours. It is an unpleasant surprise for patients to discover that they are going to remain conscious for their cataract surgery on the table in the operating room if they were assuming a general anaesthetic is used. Sedation is a controversial issue. Some units do not use it at all due to concerns that patients may be disinhibited from keeping still. Others use sedation liberally. Oral diazepam or short-acting benzodiazepines in suitable patients can be a good option, as the loss of motor control associated with IV sedation is not usually a problem. Patients who require general anaesthesia are generally those that for any reason (e.g. movement disorders, severe learning difficulties) would struggle to stay still.

Local anaesthesia is largely speaking a choice between a sub-Tenon block or topical anaesthesia. Where patients are able to keep still and are not squeezing their eyelids when having their eye examined, topical anaesthesia is a good option. It allows faster visual recovery from anaesthesia and no conjunctival scarring. However, less co-operative patients may benefit from a formal block. Note that topical anaesthesia is always topical and intracameral, not just drops alone.

Who would be appropriate to perform the surgery?

Patients with only one functioning eye should not be placed on a solo trainee list. Traumatic cataracts and white cataracts are also potentially high risk and would be better suited to a supervised list (though a trainee can still operate on these cases when experienced enough). Small pupils and floppy irises may be fine for most trainees who are operating solo to manage. However, zonule deficiencies and socially complicated patients may be more appropriate for consultant lists.

Do you need to order a special lens?

It is worth knowing what the maximum and minimum power of the lenses are that you have in your unit, as people with extremes of refraction might require lenses to be specially ordered, which can sometimes take weeks to arrive.

SUMMARY: APPROACH TO THE CATARACT CLINIC

The following is a list of important factors that include some of the areas discussed above.

Basic History

- Symptoms:
  - Can these be attributed to cataract? Typical symptoms include: glare, difficulty night driving, reading, watching television
- Past ocular history:
  - Refractive status
  - Any ocular trauma previously? This may weaken zonules
  - Any previous surgery? Actively ask if any laser refractive surgery
- Past medical history:
  - Any medical problems that cause difficulty in lying flat and still for 30 minutes, e.g. heart failure, COPD, chronic back pain
- Drug history:
  - Alpha blockers, e.g. tamsulosin, doxazosin
  - Blood thinners do not need to be stopped for cataract surgery
- Allergies:
  - Penicillin/cephalosporins in particular as cefuroxime is used as antibiotic prophylaxis
  - Skin tape
  - Preservatives in drops (may need preservative-free post-op medications)

- Social history:
    - Communication: Is an interpreter needed?
    - Who is available to help out at home, especially important in only-eye cases?
    - Any impediments to using drops? If it is tricky to use post-op steroid drops, a subconjunctival injection of dexamethasone following surgery may be a good idea

Basic Examination

- Acuity:
    - Is the acuity good enough in the fellow eye to allow for an easy recovery, or is the patient an only-eye patient who will need careful counselling prior to surgery?
    - If the eye in question has a good acuity, why is cataract surgery being considered? Is it definitely necessary?
- Face:
    - A large nose may impede a superior approach.
    - Deep set eyes are best operated on with a temporal approach.
- Lids:
    - Is there marked blepharitis or lid malposition that may pose an infection risk?
    - Are lids tight from conditions such as cicatrising pemphigoid that might make speculum insertion difficult?
- Cornea:
    - Is there significant dry eye that may be exacerbated after surgery?
    - Are there any signs of corneal ectasia that would complicate biometry calculations? (keratometry values will assist in diagnosis here)
    - Are there corneal opacities that would make surgery difficult?
    - Are there corneal guttata? A dispersive viscoelastic may be needed here to protect the endothelium.
- Anterior chamber:
    - Is there evidence of uveitis which would need to be quiet before surgery?
    - Does the anterior chamber appear shallow?

- Pupil:
  - Actively look for pseudoexfoliation on pupil margin and lens (requires dilation often).
  - Is there heterochromia suggesting Fuchs' cyclitis that may then aggressively flare after cataract surgery? This may require a pulse of IV steroid perioperatively and should be discussed with a uveitis specialist.
  - How well dilated is the pupil? Might they need mechanical pupil dilation during surgery?
- Lens:
  - How dense is the cataract?
  - Is there phacodonesis?
  - Is there posterior lens defect, e.g. from previous intravitreal injections or vitrectomy?
- Posterior pole:
  - Is there macular, optic nerve or peripheral retinal disease that is also affecting the vision, resulting in a guarded prognosis?

If there is no fundal view, then an ultrasound B Scan is advised before listing a patient for surgery.

APPROACH TO CATARACT SURGERY: THE PRE-OP "WARD ROUND"

General Approach

Everyone approaches the cataract ward round slightly differently. If you are operating with a consultant, it is worth checking with them (especially when you are very junior) whether they would prefer to conduct the ward round themselves or whether you should start this yourself. It is well worth trying to find out the week before your planned list what cases are planned and reviewing which cases look like they might be difficult and which are suitable for a trainee surgeon. This also applies more generally to subspecialty lists where you can then read up on operations you may not be familiar with prior to the surgery. Hopefully, all special lenses will have been ordered in advance. However, if they have not, you should check with theatre staff whether the lens can be obtained, and if not, then it may mean that the patient can be rescheduled in advance of having to come to hospital unnecessarily.

The pre-op ward round should really just be a check that all the essential paperwork is complete and the surgery is safe to proceed. Generally, it is not a good idea to leave things to be checked until the day of surgery.

Selecting a Lens

Check what the planned refractive outcome is first. Different supervisors have different approaches to what they like to target for emmetropia. Most target somewhere just under –0.5 dioptres. Generally having a "buffer zone" of myopia is a good idea as a hyperopic outcome is usually dissatisfying to patients as they require glasses for both reading and distance. Having said this, there are some surgeons who target 0 or even slightly plus targets, e.g. +0.05. This is probably the minority of surgeons and may well be based on their own audited refractive outcomes. Some like to go for more myopia than others, so you eventually get a feel of what your supervisor likes to target. Generally speaking, a hyperopic target is almost never desired, there will of course be exceptions but they are few and far between.

If you are early on in your training, bear in mind that your supervisor may not agree with your lens choice. It is a potential source of error to have multiple crossings-out on biometry so if you are selecting lenses, consider marking the biometry in pencil or keeping a list of which patients you think need which lens and then allowing your supervisor to mark the biometry sheet with the final choice.

CONCLUDING REMARKS

Cataract surgery may be the only operation that a patient has in their lifetime. Although it will soon become a very common operation for you to perform, do not lose sight of the significant problems that can arise from inadequate safety checks or poor communication. Make time to discuss things through with patients. Remote consultations can always be easily scheduled once the initial clinical examination has been performed. The better relationships you foster with patients, the less "demanding" or "difficult" patients you will find you encounter.

18

LOCAL ANAESTHESIA

Thomas Sherman

A great deal of ophthalmic procedures are carried out under local anaesthesia, which has the benefit of a rapid patient recovery and reduced likelihood of needing admission for post-op recovery. In this chapter we review the different methods of giving local anaesthesia and pharmacology of some of the agents used.

TOPICAL

Three drops are available as anaesthetics: proxymetacaine, oxybuprocaine (commonly referred to as benoxinate) and tetracaine (Figure 18.1). There is also a lidocaine/fluorescein minim available. The acidic pH of topical anaesthetics causes them to sting when instilled. Tetracaine has a pH of 4.54 so stings more than the less acidic proxymetacaine pH 4.64.[1] There is evidence of inhibition of bacterial growth by topical anaesthetics,[2] with tetracaine being most pronounced in this effect. Tetracaine is generally felt to be a stronger anaesthetic so is used where a more invasive procedure such as subconjunctival injection is planned, whereas proxymetacaine is adequate for short procedures such as Goldmann applanation tonometry.

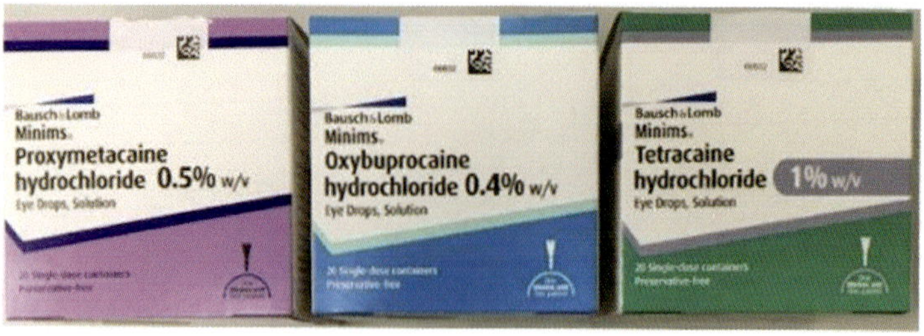

Fig. 18.1 Topical anaesthetic drops.

Their duration of anaesthesia is around 30 minutes. It is worth cautioning patients about eye rubbing/instilling contact lenses in this interval. Repeated administration of topical anaesthetic continuously for days is not encouraged as it can result in corneal epithelial breakdown.

INTRACAMERAL

Intracameral lidocaine 2% is a commonly used anaesthetic during cataract surgery. This is used as an adjunct to topical anaesthesia, which means that the patient has no conjunctiva-breaching procedure to anaesthetise the eye. This can be of benefit in situations where one is trying to limit the interference with the natural structure of the conjunctiva, for example in cases where glaucoma surgery may be planned or in ocular cicatrising pemphigoid. It is important that the anaesthetic used is preservative free (will say that the preparation is suitable for intrathecal/caudal/epidural injection) as use of preservative intracamerally can lead to an aggressive inflammatory reaction known as toxic anterior segment syndrome. A licenced preparation such as Mydrane® (Thea Pharmaceuticals Ltd.) is best used and has the added benefit of including dilating agents (tropicamide 0.02%, phenylephrine 0.31% and lidocaine 1%).

It is worth bearing in mind that a patient having topical anaesthesia will have a greater preservation of vision compared to sub-Tenon anaesthesia, which may be of benefit, for example, in only-eye cases where one wants to limit interference with vision in the short-term recovery. However, it may be necessary to reassure patients to a greater extent than with a local anaesthetic block. They will be able to see the surgeon and team members when initially taken to theatre, but after the anaesthetic is given and the procedure started, they will not see any details of the operation clearly. Using topical/intracameral anaesthesia is best used in patients who can easily relax and maintain fixation. Performing surgery on people who squeeze their lids and tend to look around a lot may be an unnecessary challenge that can be circumvented with the use of sub-Tenon anaesthesia. You can assess for this at the slit lamp by seeing how well patients tolerate having the lids separated with topical anaesthetic. Additionally, it is worth advising patients when the intracameral anaesthetic is being applied as it can cause an aching sensation. The anaesthetic will adequately treat the iris, which is the main source of discomfort in cataract surgery and can be topped up during surgery if needed.

SUBCONJUNCTIVAL

This is typically used when giving a large-calibre intraocular injection such as a dexamethasone implant (e.g. Ozurdex). The issue with giving anaesthesia subconjunctivally is that it will distort the conjunctival anatomy for judging distance from the limbus, so large volumes are best avoided. It is uncommon to use subconjunctival anaesthesia in other settings. However, it can be useful for anterior chamber paracentesis and if multiple injections are being given for endophthalmitis treatment (although in the author's opinion, a sub-Tenon block is usually better for this).

SUB-TENON BLOCK

A large proportion of cataract surgery is now performed under sub-Tenon anaesthesia, as well as other operations such as vitrectomies and some laser procedures such as cyclodiode laser treatment. In trabeculectomy surgery, the surgeon will be keen to avoid any subconjunctival haemorrhage which can result in scarring and poor outcomes, so some surgeons will opt for peribulbar anaesthesia. However, sub-Tenon's anaesthesia can still be used in this setting but avoiding large conjunctival vessels.

There are multiple techniques that can be used for giving sub-Tenon injections in general. Plain lidocaine 2% is the typical agent used. Some units give an additive called hyalase, which is believed to improve penetration of the anaesthetic and improve akinesia.[3] The traditional method of giving sub-Tenon anaesthetic with a sub-Tenon kit is as follows:

1. Check patient identification and eye to be treated.
2. Apply topical anaesthetic.
3. Apply topical iodine and clean lids.
4. Create a sterile area with a sub-Tenon kit and appropriate anaesthetic drawn up.
5. Apply a lid speculum.
6. Direct the patient to look upwards and laterally, then to grasp conjunctiva around 5 mm from the limbus inferonasally and lift slightly upwards to form a triangle.
7. Direct a pair of closed Wescott scissors through this triangle and blunt dissect to the post-equatorial region. Follow the curvature of the globe around. This means that the scissors should move from a near-horizontal to near-vertical endpoint.
8. Insert the sub-Tenon cannula through this opening and inject 2–4 mL of lidocaine.

Other techniques described for administering sub-Tenon have described using a triport sub-Tenon cannula (Eagle cannula), which can be directly inserted into sub-Tenon space without the need to dissect an opening to the space. A video demonstrating this technique can be found in the supplementary material of the article detailing the technique.[4] A 21-gauge 25 mm angled triport sub-Tenon anaesthetic cannula (Eagle Labs,

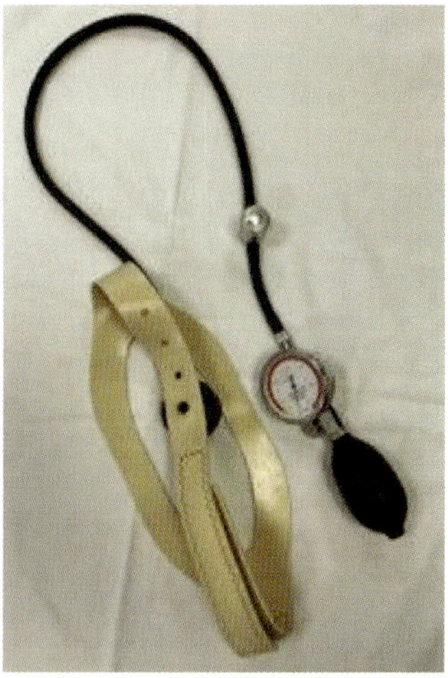

Fig. 18.2 Honan's balloon. The small black circle is placed over the eye with gauze underneath and the pressure gauge has a mark indicating the appropriate amount of inflation.

Cucamonga, CA, USA) is used for the technique. Another alternative technique is using a 20-gauge (pink) IV cannula that has the needle removed. However, this still requires introduction through an incision prepared with either scissors or an 18-gauge needle.[5]

Once the local anaesthetic has been administered, pressure is usually applied for a few minutes over the eye to ensure that the anaesthetic is distributed posteriorly. A Honan's balloon (figure 18.2) is a device available in some units which can be attached around a patient's head and inflated to provide pressure around the eye aimed at promoting posterior distribution of anaesthetic. There is a small black balloon connected to a pump similar to a blood pressure cuff which is inflated and kept on until arrival into main theatre.

Peribulbar/Retrobulbar

Peribulbar injections are used with decreasing frequency with the advent of sub-Tenon anaesthesia becoming more

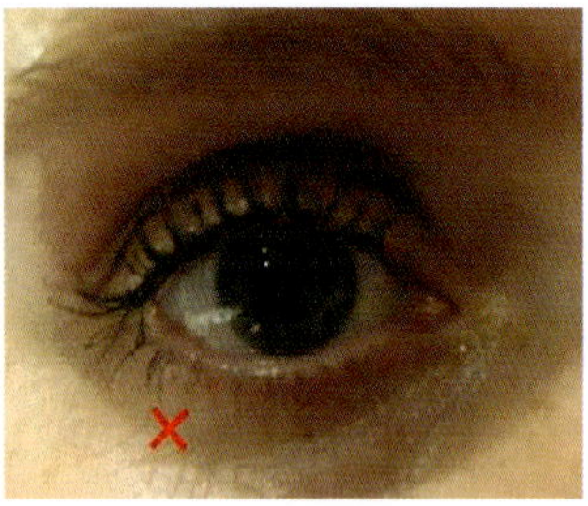

Fig. 18.3 Anatomical site for peribulbar injection (same for retrobulbar anaesthetic as well).

widespread in ophthalmic practice. However, there are some centres where they are routinely used. A peribulbar injection of local anaesthetic can be administered in multiple methods. However, perhaps the simplest is through a single inferior injection of around 5 mL given inferolaterally in a transcutaneous manner. This is sited at a point between the lateral third and medial two thirds of the inferior orbital rim (Figure 18.3).

A 2.5 mm needle is directed towards the orbital floor and aspirated as it is advanced to ensure that a blood vessel has not been entered. Then, 2–5 mL is administered, which should achieve adequate akinesia and anaesthesia. As peribulbar anaesthetic uses a sharp needle, there is a risk of globe perforation, especially in eyes with a large axial length or posterior staphyloma, so it has become less commonly used than sub-Tenon anaesthesia.

Retrobulbar injection of anaesthesia is no longer used in UK practice. Interestingly, it is still widely used in the USA and Canada. There is a small risk of damaging orbital vessels, optic nerve and even brainstem anaesthesia. Although these are rare risks, they don't occur with peribulbar and sub-Tenon injection, so these have replaced retrobulbar blocks accordingly.

Subcutaneous

This is used for lid surgery principally. Most centres will use 1% or 2% lidocaine with adrenaline (1:1000). However, other forms of anaesthesia such as levobupivacaine can be used. The

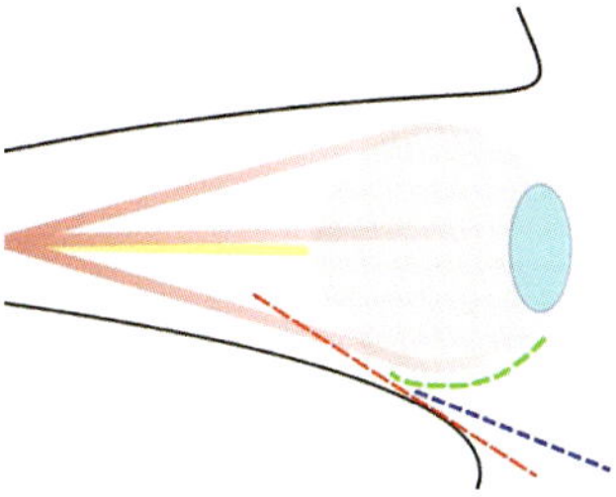

Fig. 18.4 Trajectory for different local anaesthetic blocks, green line is sub-Tenon following the globe to past the equator. Peribulbar in blue which delivers anaesthetic at the equator. Retrobulbar in red which delivers anaesthetic into the cone (note that the needle does not pass through the body of the muscle but between the recti muscles).

acidity and cold temperature of the local anaesthetic can make this an uncomfortable procedure. Warming the anaesthetic slightly can improve the comfort. The following is a technique that can also minimise discomfort:

1. Instil strong topical anaesthetic.
2. Stand behind the patient with them lying flat. Lower the lower lid and pass the local anaesthetic needle vertically downwards anterior to the orbital rim but through the conjunctival side of the lower lid. Inject the local anaesthetic.
3. The lower lid should now be reasonably numb. The superficial lid tissue can then be further anaesthetised through subcutaneous injection of the lower lid, starting medially and moving towards the lateral canthus. Make sure the lateral canthus is adequately anaesthetised.
4. Once at the lateral canthus inject under the upper lid skin, keeping the needle facing away from the globe.
5. Once subcutaneous anaesthetic has been given, the lid should be everted and just lateral to the everted lid the needle can be inserted under a small pocket of conjunctiva to provide anaesthesia of the posterior lamellae.

Take care anaesthetising the lids where ptosis and blepharoplasty procedures are planned as too much anaesthetic or bruising can disrupt the tissue planes and make surgery difficult, as well as distorting pre-operative markings. Any markings of the skin should be made before injecting local anaesthetic.

CONCLUSIONS

Local anaesthetic blocks are widely used in ophthalmology practice, approaches are summarised in figure 18.4. Being familiar with sub-Tenon anaesthesia and subcutaneous lid anaesthesia is particularly important as these are the most commonly performed local anaesthetic procedures.

References

1. Weaver CS, Rusyniak DE, Brizendine EJ, *et al.* (2003) A prospective, randomized, double-blind comparison of buffered versus plain tetracaine in reducing the pain of topical ophthalmic anesthesia. *Ann Emerg Med* **41**(6): 827–831.
2. Pelosini L, Treffene S, Hollick EJ. (2009) Antibacterial activity of preservative-free topical anesthetic drops in current use in ophthalmology departments. *Cornea* **28**(1): 58–61.
3. Rowley SA, Hale JE, Finlay RD. (2000) Sub-Tenon's local anaesthesia: the effect of hyaluronidase. *Br J Ophthalmol* **84**(4): 435–436.
4. Lin S, Ling RH, Allman KG. (2014) Real-time visualisation of anaesthetic fluid localisation following incisionless sub-Tenon block. *Eye* **28**(4): 497–498.
5. Anon. (2019) Modified Subtenon Block. American Academy of Ophthalmology. Available at: https://www.aao.org/1-minute-video/modified-subtenon-block [Accessed October 21, 2021].

19

BASIC PRINCIPLES OF BIOPSY

Sarah Levy

Eyelid lesions may be benign or malignant. Diagnosis is made based on the history, clinical examination and histology gained from biopsy. Biopsy of eyelid lesions can be divided into incisional and excisional biopsy. Deciding on which to perform is dependent on patient factors, the location and size of the lesion and clinical suspicion. Occasionally, multiple or "map" biopsies are taken to determine the extent of malignant change.

The gold standard for excision of malignant lesions in the periocular region is Mohs micrographic surgery, where the tissue is excised in layers and examined at each stage for cancer cells. This minimises the amount of tissue excised whilst ensuring complete excision of cancer cells. Mohs surgery is usually performed by dermatologists and is often a limited service. It is therefore commonly reserved for medial canthal lesions where tissue for reconstruction is limited and where ensuring complete excision is essential to avoid deeper extension into the orbit.

For all biopsies, the procedure should be performed in sterile conditions, with cleaning to the skin and sterile gloves worn. Care should be taken when handling the tissues so that the biopsy is not crushed. Most specimens are sent in formalin but if an unusual sample is being taken, discuss with the histology department as to how they would like to examine the specimen prior to surgery.

INCISIONAL

Incisional biopsies are taken to confirm a diagnosis and are taken with a blade which provides the ability to vary and control the size and shape of the biopsy. It is important to take a good depth of biopsy as cancerous cells may lie deep to superficial ulceration or keratin. A small amount of presumed normal tissue is also taken with the sample for histology purposes.

Large defects can be closed with suture whilst smaller defects can be left to heal by secondary intention.

PUNCH

A punch biopsy (Figure 19.1) is commonly used in dermatology but can be used in the periocular region. There is less control over depth and size but a punch biopsy does allow good examination of skin and dermis. A 4 mm biopsy, using a disposable punch biopsy, is standard but other sizes are available.

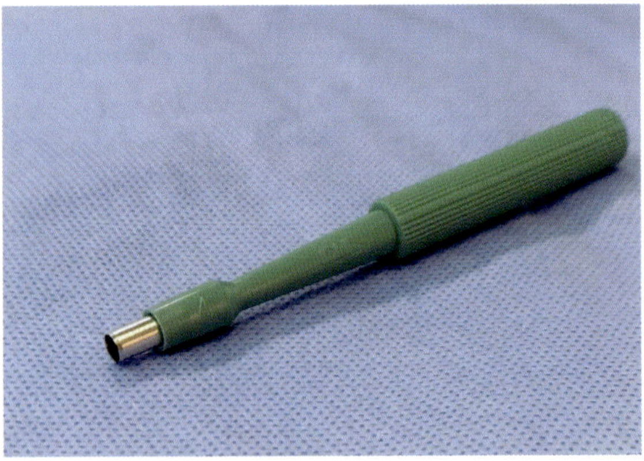

Fig. 19.1 Punch biopsy.

SHAVE

Shave biopsies are superficial and performed parallel to the skin or lid margin. They are useful for presumed superficial, benign lesions but as it is a very superficial sample this procedure is not suitable for suspected malignancies. They heal very quickly and usually just require diathermy to the base of the excised lesion for haemostasis and to reduce the chance of recurrence.

EXCISIONAL

This involves removing the whole lesion, which is then sent for histopathology. Depending on the suspected diagnosis, a margin around the lesion of clear, normal tissue is also excised. This is the ideal management if the lesion is small and the clinician is confident in the suspected diagnosis. In the lateral and central upper and lower eyelid this is commonly taken as a wedge excision.

Depending on the defect remaining, this is closed directly with a suture or left to heal by secondary intention. If a full-thickness wedge excision is taken, the defect should be closed in 2 layers, so that the anterior and posterior lamellar are closed to avoid an eyelid notch (see eyelid suturing for details).

20

BASIC PRINCIPLES OF DIATHERMY

Sarah Levy

Surgical diathermy is a tool that can be used for haemostasis or to cut tissues. The tools use the thermal effect of high-frequency, alternating current to divide tissues and coagulate blood.

Diathermy devices can be divided into monopolar and bipolar, depending on how the electrical circuit is achieved. In each device there are two modes, "cutting" and "coagulation". In "cutting" mode, where the current flows in a continuous, alternating, low-voltage pattern, the energy from the electrode vaporises the water content of the tissue. In "coagulation" mode where the current flows in a pulsed, high-voltage pattern, the energy causes thermal coagulation of the tissues.

It is important to be aware that diathermy may interfere with patient monitoring such as ECG and pulse oximetry.

MONOPOLAR DIATHERMY

With monopolar diathermy (Figure 20.1) the current flows through a probe at high density and returns via a low-current, neutral diathermy plate which is usually placed on the patient's leg.

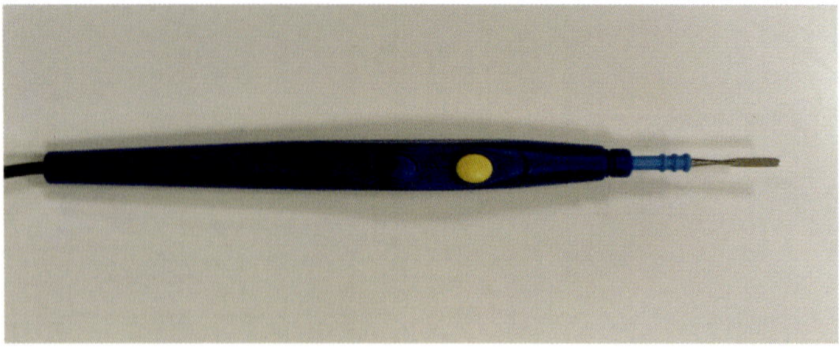

Fig. 20.1 Monopolar diathermy.

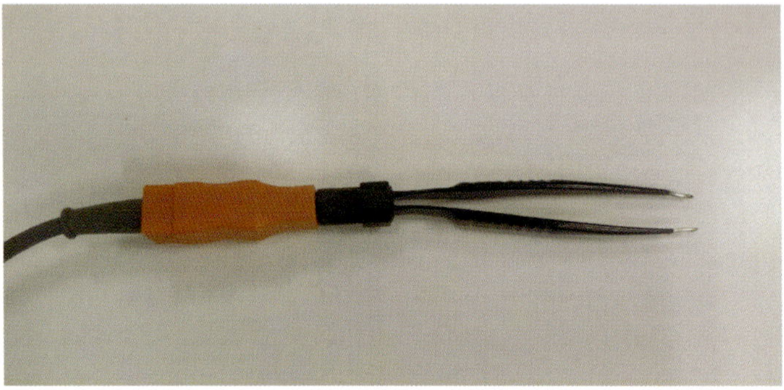

Fig. 20.2 Bipolar diathermy.

Monopolar diathermy should be avoided in patients with a pacemaker as the electrical current passing through the patient from the electrode to the diathermy pad may interfere with the pacemaker. It is important to ensure that the neutral plate is correctly attached to avoid thermal burns.

BIPOLAR DIATHERMY

With bipolar diathermy (Figure 20.2) the current flows between the two probes of the forceps. One delivers high-density current and the other completes the circuit so that the tissues between the forceps are heated. For this reason the forceps need to be held with a small distance between the probes to be effective.

21

EYELID SUTURING

Sarah Levy

The basic principles of eyelid suturing are the same for eyelid trauma as they are for wedge excision biopsy repair. The aim of eyelid suturing is to realign the eyelid margin and therefore avoid an eyelid notch (which can cause corneal abrasion and watering), restoring eyelid function (primarily, ocular surface protection). Tension should be directed parallel to the eyelid margin rather than vertically (Figure 21.1) to avoid causing lower or upper eyelid ectropion.

In cases of trauma, it is essential to carefully explore the extent of the wound, examine the canalicular system with lacrimal syringing and perform a thorough ocular examination to assess any ocular damage.

ANATOMY

It is important to have a good understanding of eyelid anatomy to ensure correct alignment. The eyelid can be divided into the anterior and posterior lamellae, divided by the grey line at the eyelid margin and the orbital septum above the tarsal plate. The anterior lamellar comprises skin and orbicularis oculi. The posterior lamellar is made up of tarsal plate and tarsal conjunctiva with the meibomian glands running within the tarsus.

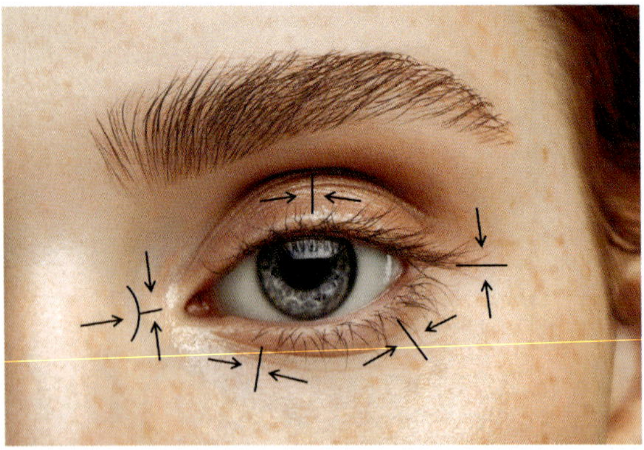

Fig. 21.1 Black lines indicating scar perpendicular to lid margin, arrows indicating the direction of force.

The levator palpebrae superioris muscle is responsible for elevating the upper eyelid. It arises posteriorly from the lesser wing of sphenoid. It forms a broad band, the aponeurosis, and inserts into the anterior surface of the tarsus.

CONSENT

Patients requiring eyelid suturing need to be consented for the following:

- Infection
- Bleeding/bruising
- Scarring
- Asymmetry
- Eyelid notch
- Watering
- Need for further surgery

PRE-OPERATIVE CHECKS

1. Confirm the identity of the patient with the notes including name and date of birth

2. Confirm that the patient has signed a consent form and that they can confirm the side of the procedure
3. Mark the correct eye

EQUIPMENT

Simple eyelid lacerations involving the skin and orbicularis may be closed with simple, interrupted sutures, with a sterile environment at the bedside. Full-thickness lacerations or lacerations involving the eyelid margin require careful alignment and are therefore better performed in the operating theatre.

- Local anaesthetic
- Toothed forceps
- Needle holder
- Diathermy
- 6.0 vicryl × 2
- 7.0 vicryl rapide
- Steristrips

TECHNIQUE FOR CLOSURE OF FULL-THICKNESS EYELID WOUNDS

1. Instill the local anaesthetic to the eyelid, typically 1% lidocaine with adrenaline 1:200,000.
2. The practitioner should wash their hands and use sterile gloves, hat, gown and mask.
3. Sterilize the area around the eye with iodine or chlorhexidine.
4. Ideally, the wound should be pentagon shaped so that there is an equal amount of tarsal plate on both sides of the wound. In trauma, freshen the wound edges but be cautious of removing tissue which may be required later.
5. The first suture is very important as it determines the alignment of the lid margin. Pass a single-ended 6.0 vicryl through the orbicularis and a good bite of the tarsal plate,

exiting at the tip of the tarsus, but not though the conjunctival surface.

6. Enter the other side of the wound in exactly the same place to ensure good alignment, through the tarsal plate and out in the orbicularis. Check the alignment and replace if needed.
7. Place this suture untied on a steristrip out of the way.
8. Place two more similar sutures in the tarsal plate and place on steristrips as you go.
9. When all the tarsal sutures have been placed, tie them, starting with the superior most suture.
10. Now align the anterior lamellar at the lid margin by passing a 7.0 vicryl rapide through the orbicularis, exiting in the grey line and then from the grey line on the other side of the wound, into the orbicularis. Tie the suture which should be buried.
11. Finally close the skin with a continuous 7.0 vicryl rapide.
12. Apply antibiotic ointment and cover with a clear shield to avoid the patient rubbing the eye. If there is significant bruising, a jelonet and double pad can be used for a few hours.

POST-OPERATIVE CONSIDERATIONS

All the sutures used are absorbable and so don't need to be removed. Keep the wound greasy with antibiotic ointment to avoid scarring and review in 4 weeks.

22

TEMPORAL ARTERY BIOPSY

Sarah Levy

Biopsy of the superficial temporal artery is performed to aid diagnosis when giant cell arteritis (GCA) is suspected. GCA is a systemic inflammatory vasculitis, occurring in patients over 50, and affects medium- to large-sized blood vessels. Ophthalmic manifestations include anterior ischaemic optic neuropathy, central retinal artery occlusion and cranial nerve palsies. It may present with a range of ocular symptoms including diplopia, transient or permanent visual loss. Systemic symptoms include weight loss, headache, scalp tenderness, jaw claudication, night sweats, loss of appetite and proximal limb weakness.

Diagnosis is clinical with the aid of inflammatory markers (estimated sedimentation rate, plasma viscosity, C-reactive protein) and temporal artery biopsy. Treatment of GCA involves long-term, tapering, oral corticosteroids. Corticosteroids have significant systemic side effects including immunosuppression and therefore histological confirmation of the diagnosis with biopsy is useful. Ultrasound scanning of the temporal and axillary arteries to aid diagnosis is becoming increasingly common, however not universal, and therefore artery biopsy remains the gold standard.

PRE-OPERATIVE CONSIDERATIONS

Patients are often started on oral corticosteroids as soon as GCA is suspected. Corticosteroids may directly affect histological signs within the artery and therefore it is essential that the biopsy is performed as soon as possible after starting treatment and certainly within 2 weeks to avoid false negative results. For this reason, it is often not possible to stop the patient's anticoagulant medication prior to surgery. The procedure is usually performed under local anaesthesia.

ANATOMY

The frontal branch of the superficial temporal artery is most commonly utilised for biopsy as it is accessible and frequently involved in GCA. The artery lies deep to the subcutaneous fat, in the superficial temporal fascia. Care needs to be taken to avoid damage to the temporal facial nerve, which runs in close proximity to the artery, slightly deeper in the temporoparietal fascia. Posterior to the temporal hairline is generally deemed to be a safe area to take the biopsy as highlighted in Figure 22.1, but even within this area, care should be taken as the anatomical course of the facial nerve may vary between patients.

Due to the nature of GCA, which histologically may "skip" some parts of the artery, it is recommended that a large enough sample of artery is taken to accurately diagnose disease histologically. Ideal biopsy length is therefore 1–2 cm.

CONSENT

Patients must be consented for the following:

- Bleeding/bruising
- Infection
- Scar (this is usually hidden behind the hairline)

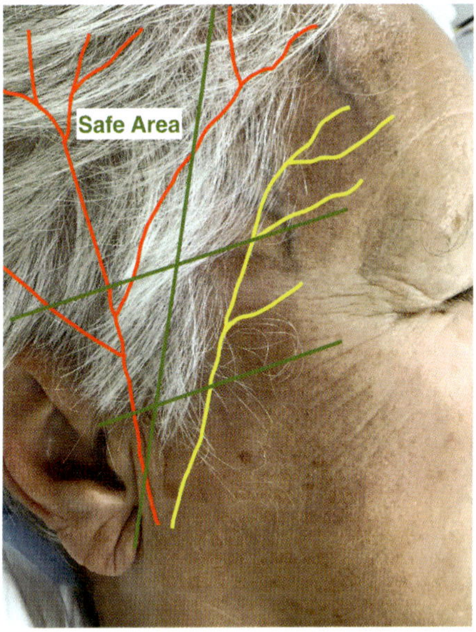

Fig. 22.1 Course of temporal artery (red), course of facial nerve (yellow), safe area for biopsy (posterior to vertical green line).

- Numbness of skin
- Scalp necrosis
- Facial weakness
- Stroke
- Need for further treatment or investigation

PRE-OPERATIVE CHECKS

1. Confirm the identity of the patient with the notes including name and date of birth.
2. Confirm that the patient has signed a consent form and that they can confirm the side of the procedure (usually the symptomatic side — headache/visual symptoms or signs) although either artery can be biopsied.
3. Mark the side for biopsy.

EQUIPMENT

General instruments include:

- Local anaesthetic
- Lid tray including blunt-ended scissors and cats paws or self-retaining retractor
- 15 blade
- Bipolar diathermy

Specific instruments:

- Electric shaver
- Handheld Doppler ultrasound
- Cataract drape
- 5.0 vicryl
- Consider 2/0 silk stay suture
- Steristrips

TECHNIQUE

1. Prior to the local anaesthetic infiltration, the course of the artery must be marked. This is done with palpation of the artery and Doppler ultrasound, particularly if the artery is difficult to palpate, which is common in GCA. The hair overlying the artery will need to be shaved.
2. Once the artery is marked, either side of the artery and in the superficial skin infiltrate with 1% lidocaine with adrenaline 1:200,000. Take care not to hit the artery as this will cause a large haematoma and make subsequent surgery difficult.
3. The practitioner should wash their hands and use sterile gloves, hat, gown and mask.
4. Sterilize the area carefully so that you do not remove the mark in the process.
5. Place the cataract drape over the marked area so that the marked artery lies in the centre of the clear window. This ensures that the hair is kept well away from the operation site (Figure 22.2).

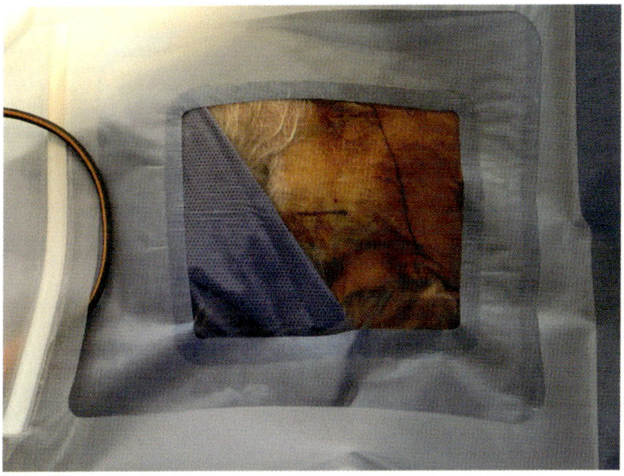

Fig. 22.2 Cataract drape over surgical site.

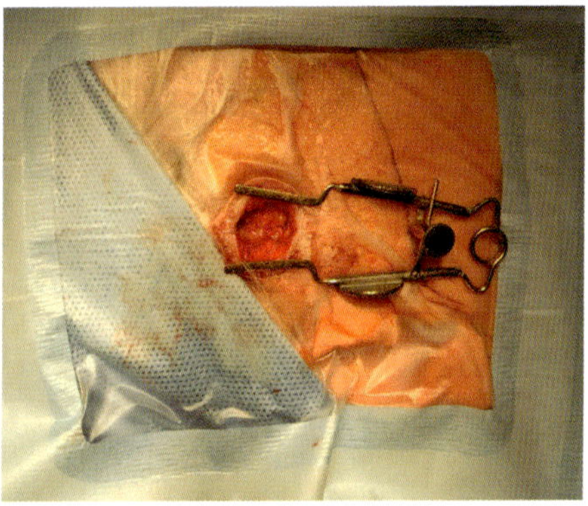

Fig. 22.3 Exposed temporal artery.

6. Make the skin incision with the 15 blade directly over the artery marked. This needs to include skin, epidermis and dermis.
7. Lift the wound edges upwards and blunt dissect the fat using blunt-ended scissors.
8. Once the artery has been identified, blunt dissection should be performed with the mosquito forceps to expose the length of the artery to be biopsied (Figure 22.3). Take care not to over-handle or crush the artery.

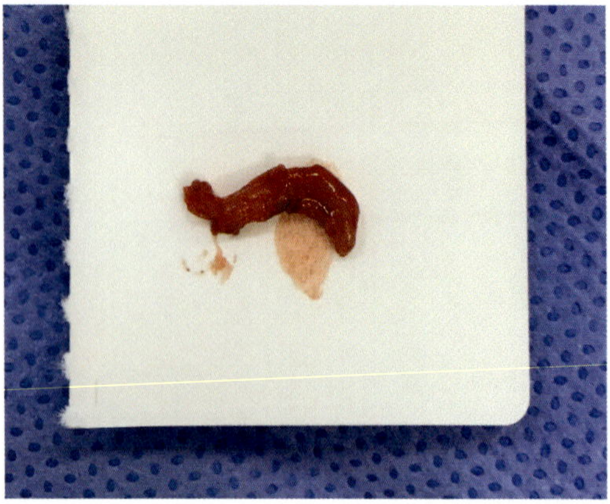

Fig. 22.4 Temporal artery specimen to be sent for histology.

9. Tie off both ends of the artery with a 5.0 vicryl. The needle can be passed with the blunt end facing forwards to reduce the risk of damaging the artery. Ensure that you have a good knot and a second can be placed if there is concern that the first is not adequate.
10. Any branches should be tied off in a similar manner.
11. Cut and remove the artery (Figure 22.4). The specimen should be placed in formalin and sent for urgent histology.
12. Close the wound with 3–4 subcuticular, interrupted, buried sutures. With good alignment this is all that is required.
13. Dress the wound with a steristrip.

POST-OPERATIVE CONSIDERATIONS

Ensure that the patient has a plan for their corticosteroid treatment and follow-up in the ophthalmology or rheumatology department.

23

CHALAZION INCISION AND CURETTAGE

Sarah Levy

CHALAZION

A chalazion is an inflammatory cyst of the meibomian gland secondary to obstruction of sebaceous secretions. The majority of chalazia are managed medically and do not require surgical treatment, with most resolving by 6 months. Patients with chalazion may present with an acute or chronic, upper or lower eyelid cyst. There may be associated pain, erythema or swelling and large chalazia may cause blurred vision. Patients may also have blepharitis or associated rosacea.

ANATOMY

The eyelid can be divided into the anterior and posterior lamellar, divided by the grey line at the eyelid margin. The anterior lamellar comprises skin and orbicularis oculi, which is responsible for eyelid closure. The posterior lamellar is made up of tarsal plate and tarsal conjunctiva with the meibomian glands running within the tarsus. There are approximately

20–25 meibomian glands running vertically in the upper eyelid, which secrete a sebaceous, lipid portion of the tear film.

MEDICAL MANAGEMENT

An acute chalazion can be treated with regular warm compress, eyelid massage and hygiene. If these measures do not improve symptoms or the chalazion is present for a number of months and still causing symptoms, incision and curettage may be required. Recurrent chalazia should be biopsied to exclude sebaceous gland carcinoma.

CONSENT

Patients need to be consented for the following:

- Infection
- Bleeding/bruising
- Scarring
- Recurrence
- Need for further surgery

PRE-OPERATIVE CHECKS

1. Confirm the identity of the patient with the notes including name and date of birth.
2. Confirm that the patient has signed a consent form and that they can confirm the side of the procedure.
3. Mark the correct eye and the location of the chalazion on the overlying skin as this can be difficult to identify once local anaesthetic has been instilled.

EQUIPMENT

Incision and curettage can be performed on a minor operations list in a sterile environment.

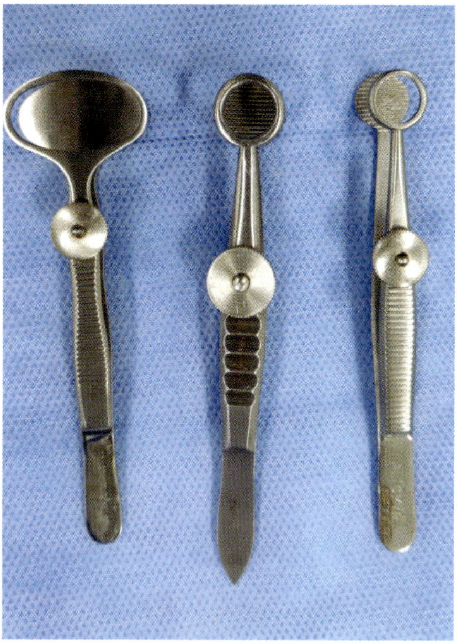

Fig. 23.1 Cyst clamp.

- Local anaesthetic
- Cyst clamp (Figure 23.1)
- 15 blade
- Curettage
- Consider diathermy
- Chloramphenicol ointment
- Double eye pad

TECHNIQUE

1. Instill the local anaesthetic to the eyelid, typically 1% lidocaine with adrenaline 1:200,000.
2. The practitioner should wash their hands and use sterile gloves.
3. Sterilize the area around the eye using iodine or chlorhexidine.
4. Place the clamp over the chalazion or marked area and tighten the clamp, so that the hole in the clamp is on the

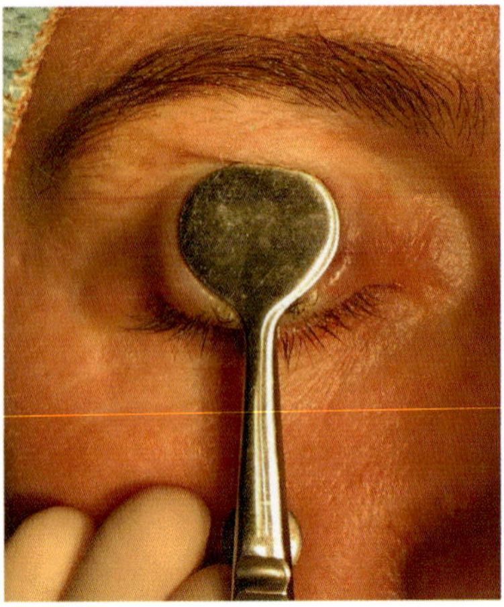

Fig. 23.2 Cyst clamp on upper lid.

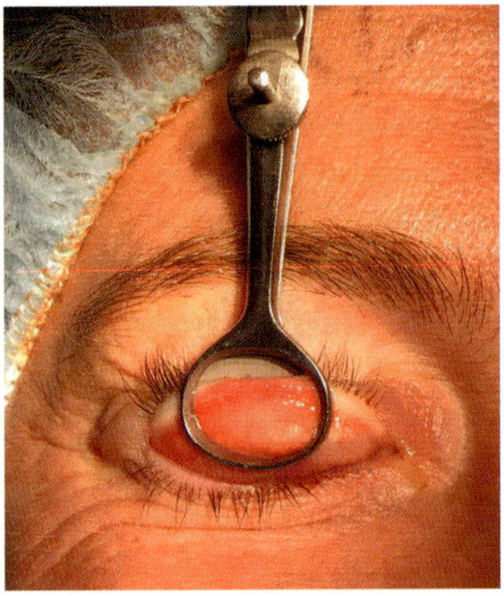

Fig. 23.3 Upper lid everted using cyst clamp.

inside of the lid and encloses the area that will be incised (Figure 23.2).

5. Use the clamp to evert the eyelid (Figure 23.3).
6. Make a vertical incision directly over the chalazion with the 15 blade (Figure 23.4). This should release pus-like material.

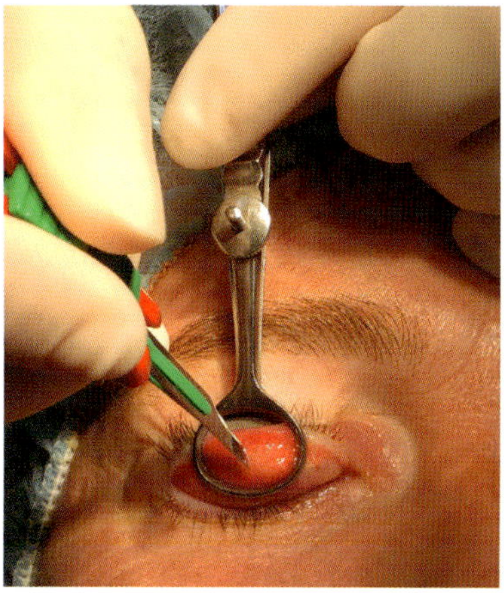

Fig. 23.4 Vertical incision over chalazion.

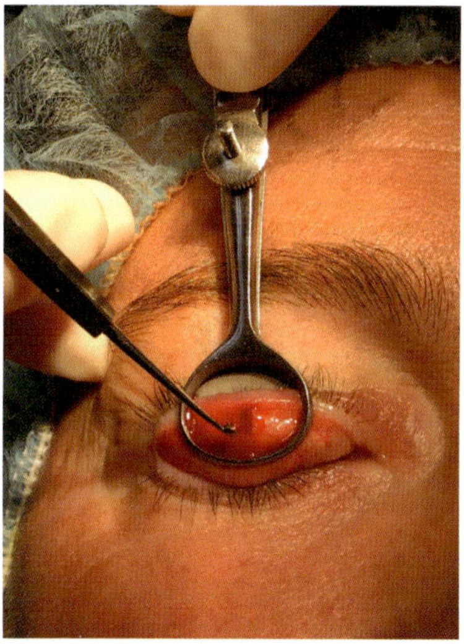

Fig. 23.5 Curettage of chalazion.

7. Curettage the wound so that the contents of the chalazion are removed (Figure 23.5).
8. At this point diathermy can be considered.

9. Instill liberal amounts of chloramphenicol ointment and double pad the eye.
10. The pad can be removed a few hours later.

POST-OPERATIVE CONSIDERATIONS

Antibiotic ointment should be prescribed for 5 days and follow-up is not usually required. Patients should be advised to perform eyelid hygiene on a regular basis to avoid recurrence.

24

ANTERIOR CHAMBER PARACENTESIS

William Spackman

INTRODUCTION

Anterior chamber (AC) paracentesis is a technique to aspirate aqueous humour from the anterior chamber of the eye. This may be necessary either as a treatment or to obtain a diagnosis.

In patients with raised intraocular pressure (IOP), AC paracentesis can quickly control the pressure, although it is not a first-line measure. In acute angle closure glaucoma, for example, initial treatment with IV acetazolamide, topical pressure lowering drops and miotic agents are often enough to reduce IOP and clear the cornea to facilitate peripheral iridotomy. IV mannitol may also be given in suitable patients as a second-line treatment. Rarely, however, IOP may be refractory to this treatment and AC paracentesis may be an option. It must be remembered that in such cases the procedure is technically very difficult as the eye is painful, the anterior chamber shallow and visualisation limited due to corneal oedema. In such a difficult case, senior help must be sought before proceeding with a paracentesis.

AC paracentesis can also be performed in patients presenting in the first few hours with central retinal artery occlusion (CRAO). The theory is that a rapid reduction in IOP from paracentesis will increase retinal perfusion and potentially dislodge an embolus. However, it is not clear how effective this is in practice.

AC paracentesis may also be performed to collect a sample of aqueous humour that can be analysed to obtain or confirm a diagnosis. This may be useful in infectious uveitis, endophthalmitis or in suspected malignancy.

PRE-PROCEDURE

Paracentesis can be performed at the slit lamp, enabling IOP control to be achieved rapidly without the need to take the patient to theatre. It is still important to maintain sterility as this is an invasive procedure with risk of intraocular infection.

In order to perform an AC paracentesis, you will need:

- Sterile gloves
- Lid speculum
- Povidone-iodine 5%
- Topical anaesthetic, e.g. tetracaine 1%
- Sterile cotton bud
- 27- or 30-gauge needle and 1 mL syringe
- Topical chloramphenicol 0.5%

Ensure that the patient is comfortably positioned at the slit lamp with their forehead resting forwards against the headrest. An assistant to support the patient may be helpful.

PROCEDURE

- Wash hands thoroughly and put on sterile gloves.
- Insert topical anaesthetic.
- Insert the lid speculum.

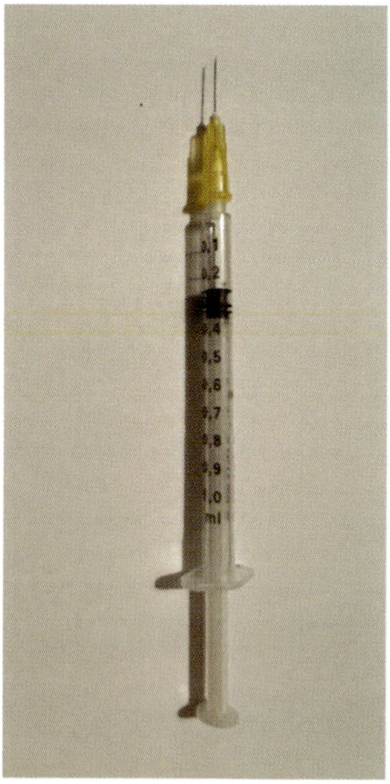

Fig. 24.1 Plunger attached to draw a sample from the AC.

- Place a drop of povidone-iodine 5% on the corneal surface.
- Soak the cotton bud in tetracaine and apply to the limbus at the area of intended insertion.
- Attach the needle to the syringe.
  - If you are performing paracentesis to lower the eye pressure, then you can remove the plunger. This will allow free flow of the aqueous humour into the syringe.
  - If you are performing an anterior chamber tap, then keep the plunger attached in order to collect the sample.
- Ensure that the patient's eye is still by giving them a target to look at such as your shoulder.
- Hold the needle and syringe in a pen-like grip with the bevel facing away from the cornea.
  - If you are performing a paracentesis on a right eye, it is best to hold the needle and syringe in your left hand and approach the cornea temporally. This ensures that the patient's nose

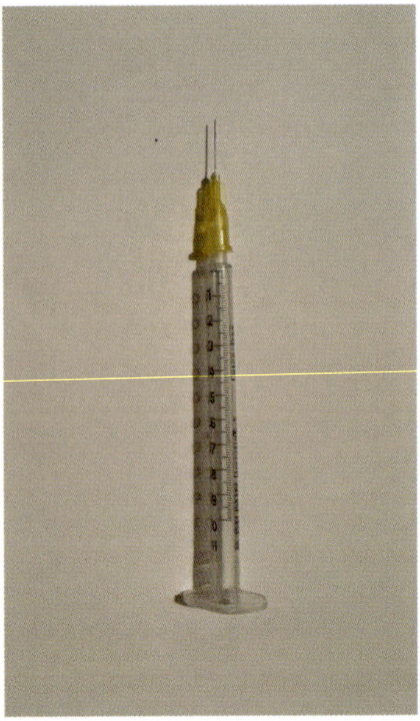

Fig. 24.2 Plunger detached to allow free flow.

does not obstruct your approach. It is important to enter the anterior chamber parallel to the iris plane.

- o If you are performing a paracentesis of the left eye, approach the cornea temporally with the needle and syringe in your right hand.

- Insert the needle at the paralimbal, clear cornea, ideally inferiorly over the iris so that you are less likely to damage the lens should the patient move or AC collapse.
  - o The needle should be inserted parallel and anterior to the iris plane.
- Insert the needle so that the whole bevel is inside the anterior chamber but do not insert any further than this to avoid inadvertent trauma.
  - o Take care to not damage the corneal endothelium, lens or iris.
- Allow some of the aqueous humour to drain from the anterior chamber until the iris begins to come forward. At this point, remove the needle.

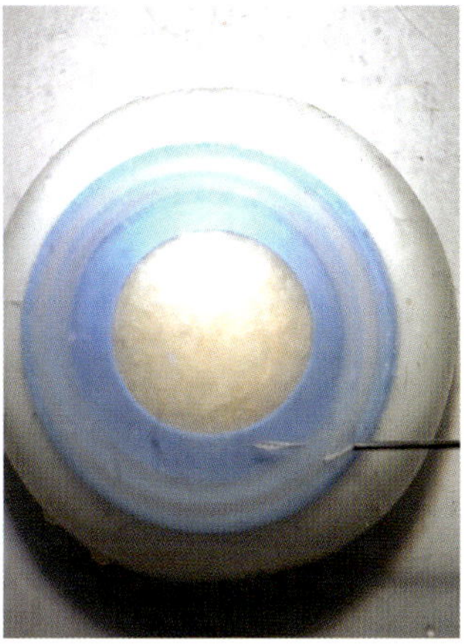

Fig. 24.3 Needle within anterior chamber.

 - o If you kept the plunger inside the syringe, withdraw in a slow and controlled manner to prevent the anterior chamber from suddenly collapsing.
- Dispose of the needle in a sharps bin.
- If sending a sample to the laboratory; place a bung on the syringe, label the sample and ensure it is delivered as soon as possible.
- Apply a drop of chloramphenicol 0.5%.
- Remove the lid speculum.

POST-PROCEDURE

- Carefully examine the anterior segment at the slit lamp to ensure that there was no iatrogenic trauma from the paracentesis.
- Give the patient a 3-day course of topical chloramphenicol as prophylaxis.
- Re-check the IOP to ensure that it is and remains adequately controlled and the eye hasn't become hypotonus.
- Further treatment may be required and paracentesis may need to be repeated if the pressure should increase again.

- In acute angle closure glaucoma, AC paracentesis may give a window in which the cornea clears to perform a peripheral iridotomy. It is important to break the cycle of angle closure, or the pressure will likely rise again.

POTENTIAL COMPLICATIONS

Performing AC paracentesis in patients with acute angle closure glaucoma may be particularly challenging. The cornea is likely to be oedematous and shallow, with impaired view of the AC. Patients may also be in some significant discomfort with pain, nausea and vomiting and remaining still on the slit lamp may be a challenge.

The most serious but rare complication of AC paracentesis is exogenous endophthalmitis. Maintaining sterility during the procedure as well as pre-procedure povidone-iodine is important to minimise the risk of this occurring.

Other potential complications include iatrogenic trauma to the cornea, iris or lens. This may result in hyphaema, cataract, infectious keratitis, or scarring.

25

AQUEOUS AND VITREOUS SAMPLING

Thomas Sherman

INTRODUCTION

Probably the most common indication for sampling of aqueous and vitreous humour is the need for culture material to diagnose infectious endophthalmitis. There are many other tests that can be performed on aqueous or vitreous humour apart from microscopy and culture. Some of these may be more specialist research investigations, while others may be used as part of more formal vitreous biopsies, e.g. to diagnose intraocular lymphoma.

In infective endophthalmitis, it is commonly advised that an aqueous/vitreous sample should be obtained within an hour. The generation time (the time taken for bacteria to double in number) is roughly 10 minutes for *Staphylococcus aureus*,[1] so prompt treatment will lessen the bacterial load within the eye. In the author's experience there are variations in practice in different units. For some, performing tap and inject procedures outside of theatre is heavily discouraged, in others it has been the norm. It is worth familiarising yourself with what tends to happen in your particular unit. Additionally, different units may use different antibiotic preparations for treating endophthalmitis, so it is worth familiarising yourself with what is used where you work (I have summarised the common treatments at the end of this chapter).

In this chapter we will review techniques for aqueous and vitreous sampling and then discuss how to prepare commonly used antibiotics for intravitreal use.

AQUEOUS SAMPLING

A diagnostic aqueous tap is usually safe to perform outside of a theatre setting. However, steps need to be taken to minimise the risk of infection or lens touch. Lens touch especially is a problem as it will induce cataract and compromise the integrity of the anterior capsule. Iris touch is undesirable; however, it usually, at worst, leads to self-limiting iris bleeds. Removing around 0.1–0.2 mL of aqueous humour is sufficient.

Required equipment: Slit lamp, orange needle (25G), 1 mL syringe, syringe bung. A speculum is not necessary but can be useful for patients who are prone to attempting eye closure during the procedure.

Technique:

1. Apply strong topical anaesthetic, e.g. tetracaine. Consider a subconjunctival injection of anaesthetic if struggling to tolerate topical anaesthetic. Sub-Tenon blocks are not usually required.
2. Apply iodine to the conjunctiva, clean eyelids if especially dirty/marked blepharitis. Allow 3 minutes for iodine to sterilise the conjunctival fornices.
3. Clean hands and assemble needle and syringe in a sterile manner. There are a couple of approaches to obtaining aqueous humour in a syringe:
    a. The plunger can be completely removed from the syringe and pressure applied on the globe at the time of taking the paracentesis. The syringe will passively fill.
    b. Alternatively, the plunger can be left *in situ* (which reduces risk of contents spilling). However, caution is

needed that the vacuum induced when the plunger is withdrawn is not too forceful as to cause anterior chamber collapse. Moving the plunger back and forth before entering the eye allows the plunger to move slowly and with control when sampling.

4. Ensure that the patient is adequately positioned and is advised to keep their forehead against the bar of the slit lamp at all times. Have a low threshold to ask an assistant to steady the head if the patient is leaning back a lot.
5. You can use forceps, e.g. Hoskins to grasp the conjunctiva in order to provide counter traction. The conjunctiva should be grasped on the opposite side form the intended entry site. This is not essential provided the needle is carefully introduced into the anterior chamber.
6. Slowly introduce the needle into the anterior chamber, keeping parallel to the iris plane and aiming away from the pupil/lens; have the lumen pointing upwards (Figure 25.2).
7. Once you can see the needle lumen completely in the anterior chamber either:
   a. Draw the plunger back slowly by extending your index finger away from the eye (as shown in Figure 25.1).

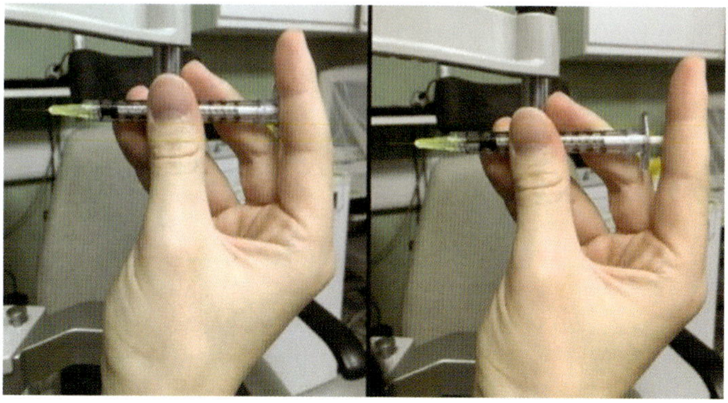

Fig. 25.1 Holding the syringe between your thumb and remaining fingers and stabilising your hand against the slit lamp, you can then move your index finger outwards to slowly and with control retract the plunger.

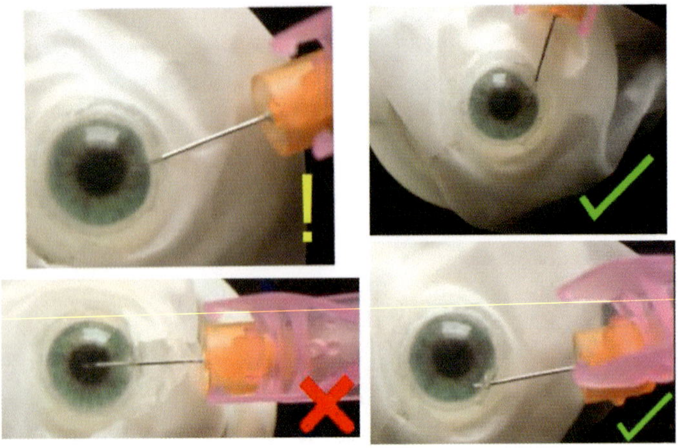

Fig. 25.2 When performing an anterior chamber tap, it is crucial to avoid the lens. In the top-left picture, the needle tip is sheltered away from the lens by iris. However, this is still risky as pushing the needle too far will result in the image below with the needle over the pupil. The right-hand images are much safer. By entering the AC lower, the needle trajectory is not going anywhere near the pupil, even if sudden further entry occurs. The same applies when the needle is directed from a superior tangent. A short-length needle as shown here is optimal for safety.

   b. If the plunger has been removed it may passively fill or gentle pressure to the opposite limbus can be applied to encourage filling.

8. When a sample has been obtained, withdraw the needle and replace with a bung to secure the sample; safely dispose of the needle in a sharps bin.
9. Provide chloramphenicol drops (or alternative topical antibiotic) to use for a week.

Given the invasiveness of acquiring the sample, it is best to ensure that the sample is hand delivered to the laboratory.

Often an anterior chamber tap is done at the same time as a vitreous tap, which may be done in theatre. Taking a patient to theatre purely for an anterior chamber tap is not often required.

In theatre you can potentially be more liberal with acquiring a sample under the operating microscope. You can create a small paracentesis using an orange needle or MVR blade, then use a Roycroft cannula attached to a 1 mL syringe to acquire the sample. This has the advantage of no sharp end inside the anterior chamber. Additionally, you can potentially acquire a larger sample of aqueous humour and refill the anterior chamber with balanced salt solution (BSS) if the anterior chamber shallows. If you are then proceeding to a vitreous chamber tap, you can ensure that the eye is firm to aid port insertion.

Vitreous Tap

Vitreous taps generally have a lower yield than anterior chamber taps, as the ease of aspiration depends on how much vitreous liquefaction has occurred. There are two main approaches to vitreous sampling, either with a syringe and needle or using a vitrector in theatre. For both, around 0.5–1 mL of vitreous can be safely removed.

Needle and Syringe Tap

Required equipment: Blue needle, 1 mL syringe, speculum, calliper, cotton bud, topical tetracaine (+/– sub-Tenon set) and iodine.

1. Sub-Tenon anaesthesia is the best form of anaesthesia for a vitreous tap. Although a conjunctival or topical anaesthetic can be used, conjunctival anaesthetic can distort the sites for injection and topical anaesthesia may not provide enough effect.
2. Apply topical iodine and allow this to sterilise the conjunctiva for 3 minutes.
3. Insert a lid speculum.
4. Ask the patient to look down and towards their nose to inject the superotemporal quadrant (a superior quadrant should be used and superotemporal is usually easiest).
5. Mark with callipers an area 3.5 mm or 4 mm posterior to the limbus if the patient is pseudophakic or phakic, respectively.

6. Displace the conjunctiva with a sterile cotton bud.
7. A blue needle attached to a 1 mL syringe is inserted perpendicular to the sclera with the direction of insertion being towards the optic nerve head; do not advance the needle fully into the eye.
8. Attempt aspiration, if the tap is dry do not repeatedly tug on the vitreous, instead ensure that the plunger is fully depressed and withdraw.

Again, these samples are precious, and so hand delivering them to a laboratory is usually the best approach.

Single Port Vitrectomy

Required equipment: 23G/25G (orange/green) vitrectomy port, vitrectomy machine, 3-way tap, 1 mL syringe, cotton swabs, drape and speculum, operating microscope.

Setting up the vitrector (a nurse is needed to assist with this):

1. Connect vitrector pneumatic driver to the machine (black tubing with grey and black ends).
2. Ensure that there is no fluid in the aspiration tubing by pressing the foot pedal whilst the probe is covered.
3. Attach a 3-way tap to the aspiration tubing (blue tubing).
4. Attach a 1 mL syringe to the 3-way tap and turn the tap "off" to this section (as shown in Figure 25.3A).
5. Set cut rate at highest rate on the machine.

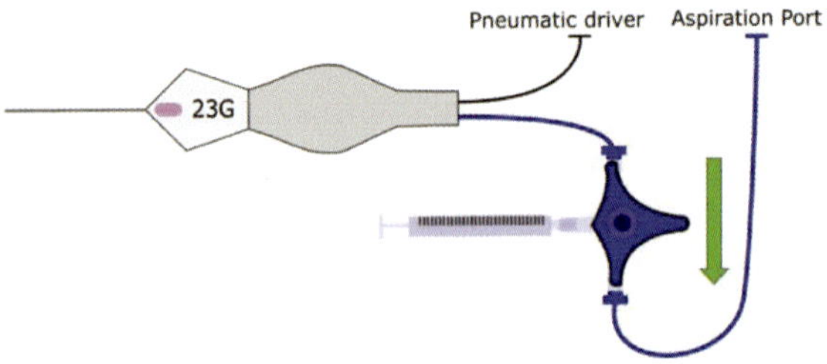

Fig. 25.3A Position of 3-way tap whilst cutting vitreous.

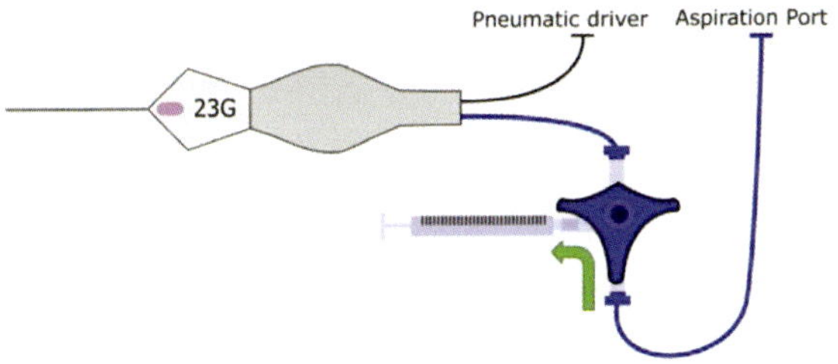

Fig. 25.3B Aspiration of distal tubing.

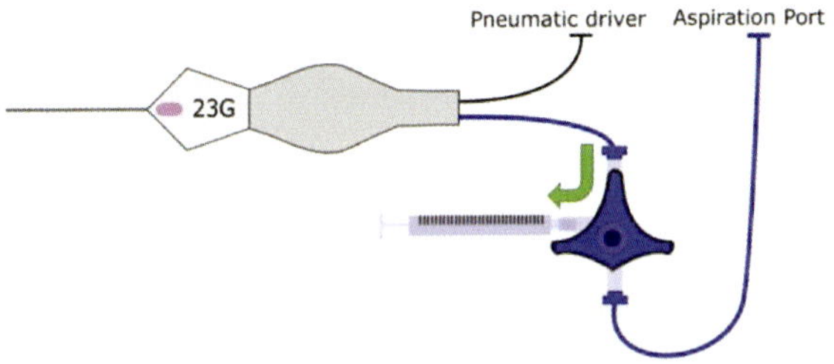

Fig. 25.3C Aspiration of proximal tubing.

Vitreous Tap

1. Sub-Tenon anaesthesia is the best form of analgesia for this procedure.
2. Standard iodine prep and cataract drape with speculum.
3. Use callipers to measure 3.5 mm or 4 mm posterior to limbus; it is usually easiest to insert the port in the superotemporal quadrant.
4. Displace the conjunctiva with forceps, e.g. Hoskins.
5. Introduce the port into the eye, with the bevel facing down, at a 30° angle initially, then re-orientate the port so it is perpendicular to the sclera once inserted about midway. This will create a stepped self-sealing entry site. Rolling the cannula back and forth between your fingertips can aid its advancement.
6. Release the trochar from the port using forceps if necessary.

7. Insert the vitrector; ensure that you are cutting whilst introducing to minimise traction on the retina, you should have the mouth of the cutter facing upwards.
8. The cutter can be visualised as a shadow behind the lens; ensure that the cutter is pointing towards the direction of the optic nerve head and gently move it to obtain vitreous.
9. Ask the nurse to inform you when clear fluid can be seen just beyond the 3-way tap.
10. Once vitreous can be seen in the tubing just past the 3-way tap, there should be enough sample to be retrieved; withdraw the cutter whilst still cutting to prevent tugging on vitreous.
11. Any drugs to be administered can be done so at this point.
12. The port is then removed from the eye with forceps, pressure applied to the entry site with cotton swab and any leak observed for.
13. If a leak is present, a single 10-0 vicryl scleral suture can be placed.
14. The sample can now be harvested from the tubing.
15. Turn the 3-way tap to the "off" position facing the cutter and aspirate the contents of the distal tubing.
16. Then turn the 3-way tap to the "off" position facing the distal tubing to aspirate the proximal tubing; you may require a second syringe to obtain all the material.
17. Place a bung over the syringe to seal container.
18. The patient can have a clear shield over their eye and topical chloramphenicol for a couple of weeks.

The advantage of using the vitrector is that there is reduced traction placed on the vitreous body when aspirating, and the yield is higher. Additionally, instead of multiple injections, one can easily give all required intravitreal injections through a single port. It does, however, necessitate more equipment to be set up and theatre time. Although this can be performed in phakic patients, you must take great care when inserting the cutter not to touch the posterior lens surface.

An alternative technique that can be used in theatre is to create a small conjunctival peritomy superotemporally; measure 3.5 mm or 4 mm depending on lens status from the limbus and create a small 80% thickness scleral flap. When this flap is lifted, multiple injections can be performed through the flap base, then the flap can be replaced and sutured down. The conjunctiva is then sutured back to the limbus. The advantage here is less need for equipment and a good seal around the site of multiple injections; however, it does require familiarity with scleral flap creation.

COMMON ANTIBIOTICS AND PROCEDURE FOR DILUTING

These doses are taken from the Moorfields Eye Hospital pharmacy accessed February 2022. Always check the expiry date of any drug to be diluted. When diluting drugs, you can use a bleed needle (small-gauge needle inserted into the vial) to break the vacuum, or aspirate the air in the powder vial to allow volume to be added easily.

Vancomycin 1 mg/0.1 mL

Beware that vancomycin has been known to cause a haemorrhagic retinal vasculitis in high doses.

1. Comes as 500 mg powder
2. Add 8 mL sodium chloride 0.9%
3. Withdraw into a 10 mL syringe and make up to 10 mL with more sodium chloride (50 mg/mL)
4. Withdraw 1 mL of this solution into a 5 mL syringe, add 4 mL sodium chloride (10 mg/mL)
5. 0.1 mL of this will give 1 mg

Ceftazidime 2 mg in 0.1 mL

1. Comes as either a 500 mg or 1 g powder
2. 500 mg powder is diluted with 4 mL water for injection
3. Withdraw entire vial into a 5 mL syringe and make up to 5 mL with sodium chloride 0.9% (100 mg/mL)

4. Withdraw 1 mL of this into a 5 mL or 10 mL syringe and make up to 5 mL (20 mg/mL)
5. 0.1 mL of this solution is withdrawn to give 2 mg

Amikacin 0.4 mg per 0.1 mL

1. Comes as a solution (500 mg/2 mL)
2. Withdraw 2 mL from the vial
3. Make up to 10 mL with sodium chloride 0.9% (50 mg/mL)
4. Shake well and discard 9 mL
5. Transfer the 1 mL into another 10 mL syringe, add 9 mL sodium chloride (5 mg/mL)
6. Draw up 8 mL of this into a sterile vial
7. Add 2 mL sodium chloride 0.9% to this vial (4 mg/mL)
8. 0.1 mL gives 0.4 mg

CONCLUSIONS

Anterior and vitreous chamber taps often occur unexpectedly and in an acute setting, it is therefore important to be familiar with the approach so you can be ready if a case of endophthalmitis suddenly presents out of hours. Intravitreal drug dilution is notoriously time consuming and prone to errors due to all the steps. Be familiar with your centre's resources and ask a nurse to double-check concentrations with you if you are a novice to drug dilution. Be aware that intravitreal antibiotics have narrow therapeutic windows and take care when diluting. Check your local formulary in case different antibiotics are advised from those listed here.

References

1. Barry P, Cordovés L, Gardner S. (2013) ESCRS Guidelines for Prevention and Treatment of Endophthalmitis Following Cataract Surgery: Data, Dilemmas and Conclusions.

Available at: https://www.escrs.org/endophthalmitis/ [Accessed February 20, 2022].

2. Han DP, Wisniewski SR, Wilson LA, *et al.* (1996) Spectrum and susceptibilities of microbiologic isolates in the Endophthalmitis Vitrectomy Study. *Am J Ophthalmol* **122**(1): 1–17.

SECTION IV
INVESTIGATIONS

26

OPTICAL COHERENCE TOMOGRAPHY

Thomas Sherman

INTRODUCTION

Optical coherence tomography (OCT) scans are the most requested ophthalmic imaging. They provide a non-invasive way of characterising the anatomy of the eye to histological-level detail. In this chapter we discuss the basic science underpinning OCT scanning and how to interpret OCT scans of the optic disc and macula. We will also briefly touch on anterior segment OCT, which is less commonly requested as well as OCT angiography.

DEVELOPMENT AND TERMINOLOGY

Prior to OCT scanning, detailed examination of the macula necessitated the use of a macular contact lens, which was applied to the patient's eye with an artificial tear coupling medium to provide a detailed view of the macula. These have now been entirely replaced with OCT.

OCT is often thought as being equivalent to ultrasound scanning using light instead of sound. The time delays in light reflections are used to judge tissue density. The early forms of OCT were termed time-domain OCTs. They relied on a reference arm mirror that physically moved, so image acquisition took more time and were of lower quality. This was superseded by spectral domain OCT in which the moving mirror was replaced by a spectrometer to detect differences in the spectral reflection of light. Enhanced depth imaging is a modification on spectral domain OCTs, where the machine is positioned closer to the retina than usual. It obtains an inverted image which visualises the choroid in more detail.

Newer OCT technology exists, termed swept source OCT. This uses a long-wavelength laser to achieve better imaging of the choroid and faster image scan times.

All of these techniques use the interferometry principle where a light source is split into a reference arm and sample arm. Reflected light produces an interference pattern that is compared to the reference arm to then make inferences about sample structure. This is demonstrated in Figure 26.1.

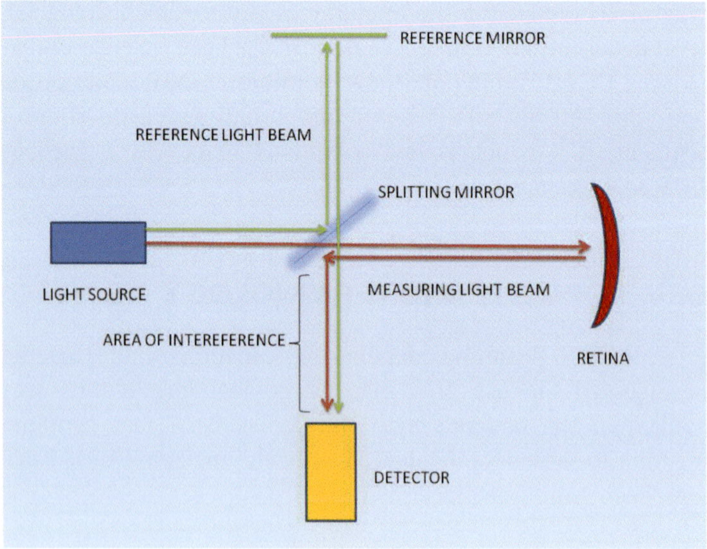

Fig. 26.1 A schematic diagram of an OCT scanner.

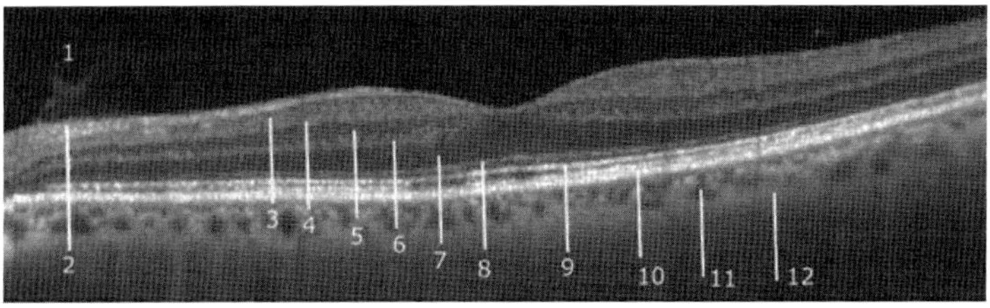

Fig. 26.2 Normal macular anatomy: (1), vitreous; (2), retinal nerve fibre layer; (3), ganglion cell layer; (4), inner plexiform layer; (5), inner nuclear layer; (6), outer plexiform layer; (7), outer nuclear layer; (8), external limiting membrane; (9), ellipsoid zone; (10), retinal pigment epithelium (RPE); (11), choriocapillaries; (12), sclera.

INTERPRETATION OF IMAGES: MACULAR OCT

A normal OCT is shown in Figure 26.2 with the normal layers of the retina labelled. Note that the thick retinal nerve fibre layer can be seen on one side of the scan, which can provide a way of determining laterality of the scan.

Describing Pathology Location

One of the most important pathological changes is the presence of retinal fluid, which can signify active neovascular disease or cystoid macular oedema requiring treatment.

Figure 26.3 shows the difference between intraretinal and subretinal fluid. Intraretinal fluid is contained entirely within the neurosensory retina itself. This is seen in post-operative CMO (cystoid macular oedema), diabetic maculopathy in particular, and is also a feature of retinal angiomatous proliferations (RAP lesions), a type of neovascular membrane that is under the age-related macular disease umbrella.

Subretinal fluid is seen between the neurosensory retina and the RPE. It could indicate an active choroidal neovascular membrane, a retinal detachment or small collections can also be seen in cystoid macular oedema (as is the case in Figure 26.3).

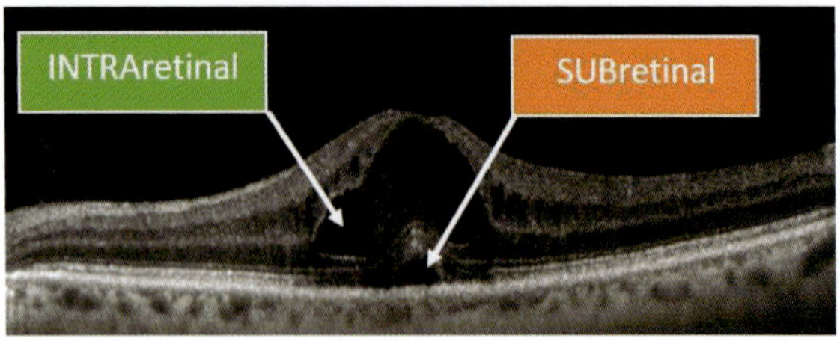

Fig. 26.3 A case of post-operative cystoid macular oedema where there is both intra- and sub-retinal fluid.

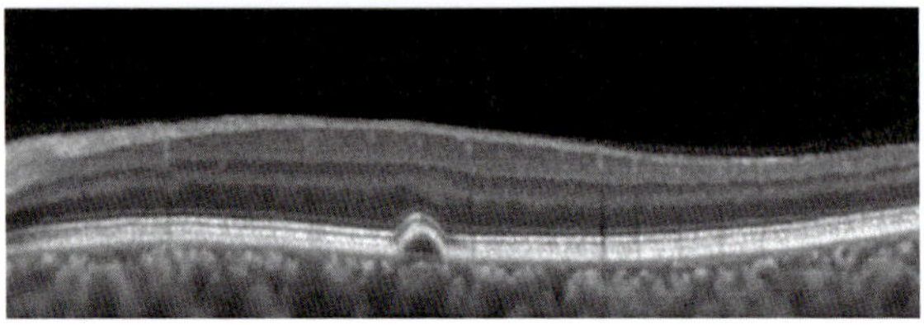

Fig. 26.4 Serous PED.

Pigment Epithelial Detachments (PEDs)

These are sub-RPE and may be drusenoid, serous or vascular in nature. Drusenoid PEDs are essentially just drusen (accumulations of lipofuscin seen in age-related macular disease). Serous PEDs are like that shown in Figure 26.4. They have a clear internal structure. These usually are associated with central serous chorioretinopathy. Vascular PEDs are usually irregular shaped and have a fibrotic component which shows as hyperreflective material under the RPE.

Technical Considerations

Most commonly, a macular scan consists of a grid of rasters (lines of pixels) in a square configuration. However, you can change the orientation of the rasters. The default setting is to use horizontal rasters. However, vertical rasters can also be selected. Sometimes doing a vertical OCT slice can be helpful when you are investigating a person with a posterior staphyloma, which can distort the OCT image (as seen in Figure 26.5).

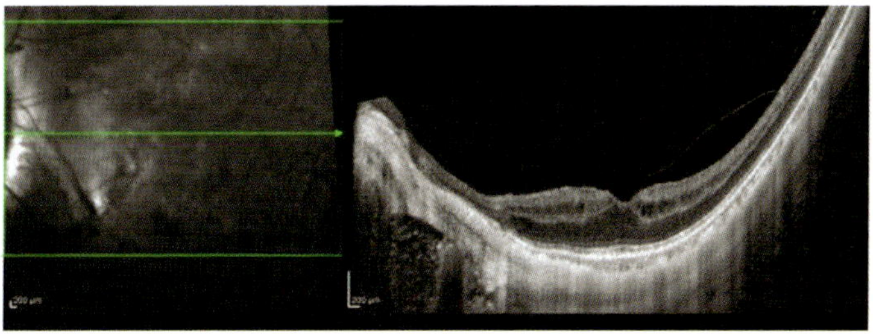

Fig. 26.5 A scan through a highly myopic eye. Note the sharp curvature of the sclera. This is due to a staphyloma being present.

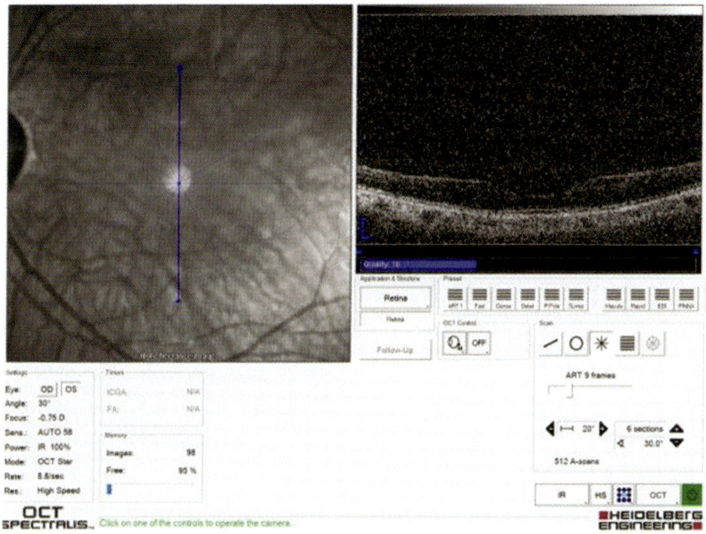

Fig. 26.6 Interface when performing an OCT scan on Heidelberg Spectralis. The bottom-right panel shows the different raster configurations, including a circular scan selected here.

Patients with high refractive error (particularly high myopia and high astigmatism) often have OCT scans that do not display as nice, flat, easy-to-interpret images. In some cases, the quality of the image can be improved by the patient keeping their glasses or contact lenses in.

Another useful setting is for taking a circular scan (Figure 26.6). This is particularly useful in trying to characterise

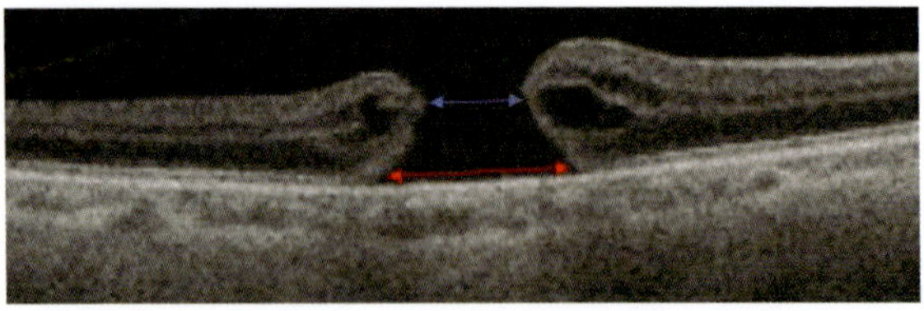

Fig. 26.7 Macular hole with measurements: MLD is the smallest distance in the OCT slice with the widest hole dimension (blue arrow). The red arrow shows the base diameter.

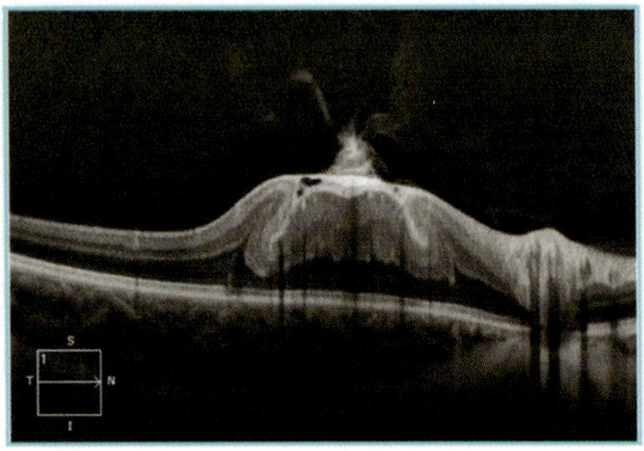

Fig. 26.8 A high-definition macular OCT showing detailed attachment of vitreous to a combined retinal hamartoma. The SD-OCT is able to show the detailed nature of the vitreous attachment and changes in the inner retinal layers.

macular holes, as the rasters are orientated in the same configuration as the pathology itself. When presented with a macular hole, the surgical management and prognosis is influenced by the base diameter and minimum linear diameter (MLD), as well as whether a PVD is present or not. These can be measured on OCT with a calliper tool. Figure 26.7 shows where these are measured from. Small holes are defined as MLD of <250 µm, medium as 251–400 µm and large as >400 µm.

Some machines (for example the Zeiss Cirrus) have a high-definition option that can be used for macular and disc OCTs. This sharpens the distinctions between retinal layers so

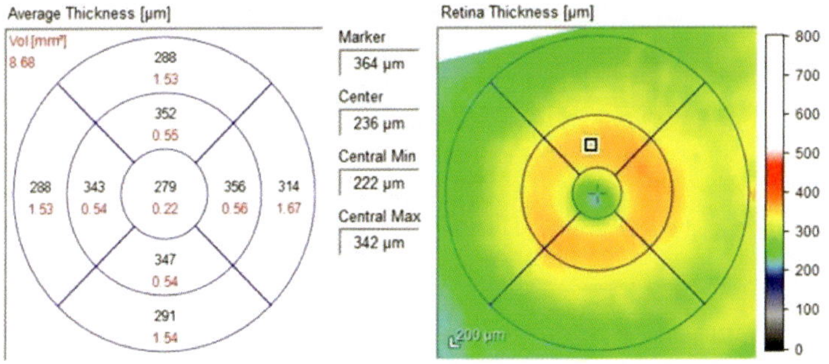

Fig. 26.9 Macular thickness cube.

is useful for characterising pathology. However, it takes fewer scans than a conventional macular grid, so is less useful for screening purposes.

Central Macular Thickness

This is a key parameter that is often used to gauge response to treatment such as intravitreal injections. It will appear as the central reading, e.g. 279 in Figure 26.9. A central macular thickness of >400 μm is of particular relevance as this is taken as a threshold for cost-effectiveness of treating diabetic macular oedema with anti-VEGF agents.

INTERPRETATION OF IMAGES: DISC OCT

OCT scans of the disc are principally used for investigating and managing glaucoma. A detailed description of interpreting disc OCTs is provided in our other book "Fundamentals of Glaucoma". However, the disc OCT can also be used in neuro-ophthalmic settings. Disc OCT provides a more effective way of documenting change from baseline in both settings rather than relying on photographs and drawings. There are three types of OCT scan that are considered as part of optic nerve head imaging:

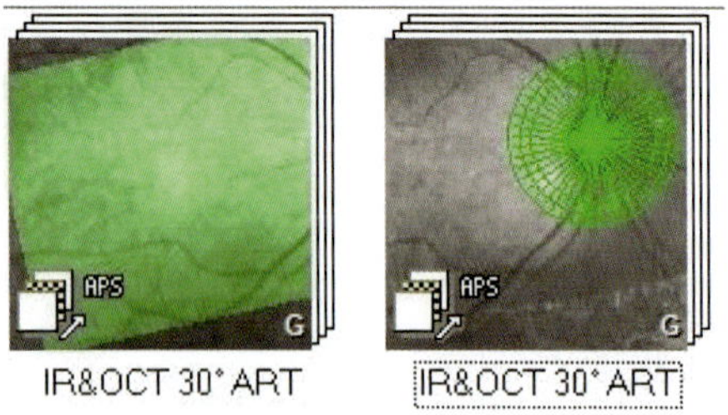

Fig. 26.10 The Heidelberg system shows the horizontal macular scan for ganglion cell thickness and the disc/peripapillary nerve fibre layer scan which is taken separately.

- Optic disc OCT
- Peripapillary nerve fibre layer OCT
- Macular ganglion cell layer OCT

Oftentimes, when a "disc OCT" is needed, it is actually all three scans that are required. So be mindful that if you are looking to investigate glaucoma, you will need a macular scan to detect a macular ganglion cell defect (just scanning the disc will not automatically scan the macula as well, Figure 26.10).

Problems With Disc OCT Interpretation

There are caveats with disc OCTs. They can be more sensitive to scan artefacts and inter-visit variation than macular OCTs. Additional issues are in interpreting the results, which are compared against a normative database kept within the machine. This database varies on the machine used, so a Heidelberg database is different from a Zeiss database. OCTs of the disc are much less reliable in high myopes and tilted discs, and can also be affected by peripapillary atrophy and vitreous attachment to the disc.

Interpreting Disc OCT Displays

In most cases, examining disc OCTs is either with a view to diagnosing/monitoring glaucoma or examining for optic disc swelling. In our other title (Fundamentals of Glaucoma) we

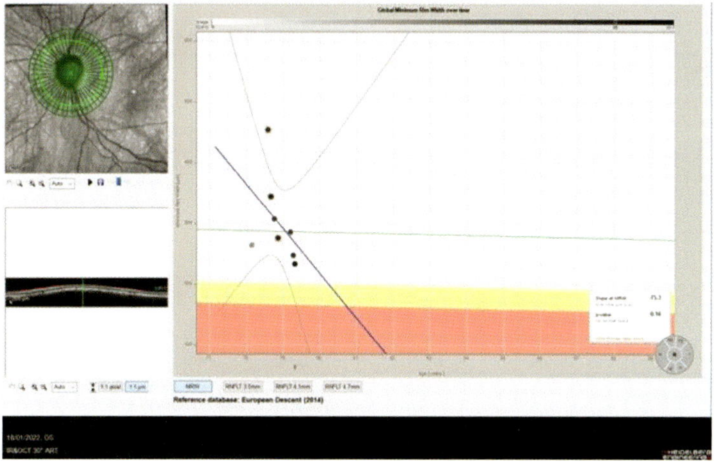

Fig. 26.11 Graph of changes in retinal nerve fibre layer thickness. This patient sustained an acute ischaemic optic neuropathy causing disc swelling, which later resolved when their blood pressure was adequately treated. Although the disc only appeared mildly swollen, you can easily see the dramatic changes in retinal nerve fibre layer thickness on this disc progression graph.

discuss more about the specific parameters to think about when examining disc OCTs in a glaucoma context. Thinking more broadly, atrophy/attenuation of retinal nerve fibres or oedema and swelling are the two main pathological processes we are interested in that OCT can help us to assess.

Once an OCT of the disc has been obtained, the differences between the patient's results and the databases are displayed in a traffic light style display (Figures 26.12 and 26.13). Note this is geared more towards diagnosing atrophy of the retinal nerve fibre layer rather than examining increasing thickness of the optic nerve head. Although swollen nerves can show up as being above the green shaded area on the disc diagram, they then tend to occupy a vague white area off the scale of measurement. It is, however, still useful to obtain a disc OCT when monitoring swelling, as it will be able to detect if there has been a decrease in thickness that may be difficult to detect on fundoscopy (Figure 26.11).

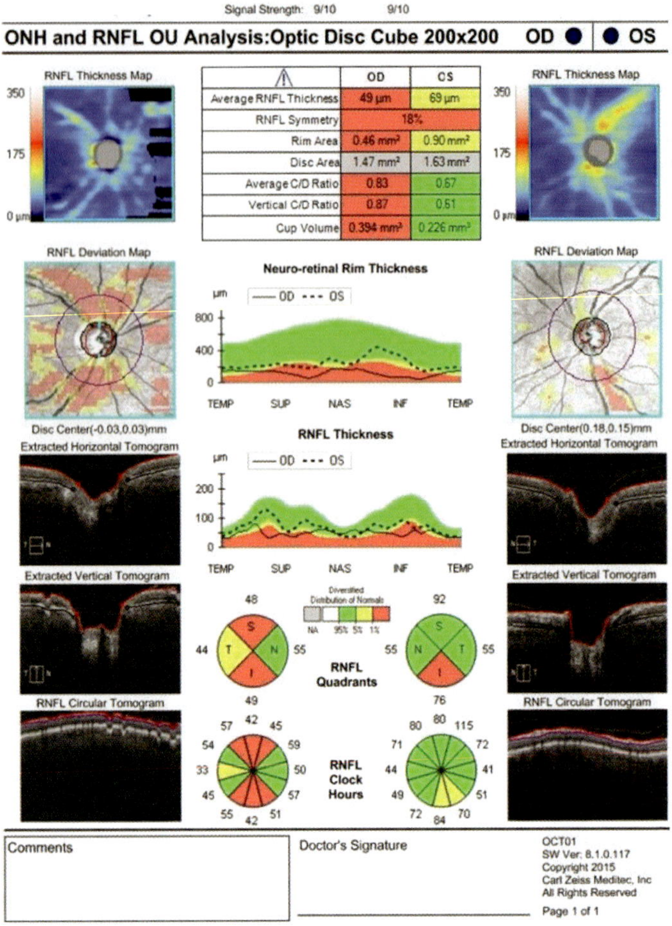

Fig. 26.12 Zeiss OCT optic disc cube display.

Approach to Interpreting Disc OCTs

This does depend on what question you are looking to answer with the OCT. However, a general approach is:

1. Check demographics and date of the scan.
2. Check accuracy: Is there blink artefact? Is there peripapillary atrophy or disc tilt that may mean a scan is inaccurate? An accuracy score is usually given for each scan and sometimes if you see a sudden dip in the profile of the retinal nerve

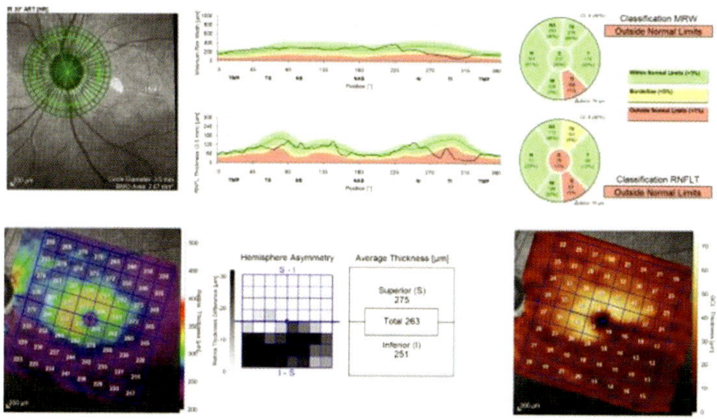

Fig. 26.13 Heidelberg glaucoma workplace display, includes macular ganglion cell analysis, which is performed separately on Zeiss machines, as shown in Figure 26.11.

fibre layer, it may mean that there has been a segmentation error.

3. Check heat maps: Are there obvious differences between eyes? For example, Figure 26.11 shows a very poor heat signal in the right eye compared to the left. In Figure 26.12 you can see a clear defect in the inferior macular area on the ganglion cell heat map in the macular region.
4. Check numeric data: Is there evidence that a "floor effect" has been reached? This is typically seen at 50 μm average retinal nerve fibre layer thickness. Beyond this point, OCT struggles to detect further thinning of the retinal nerve fibre layer and may falsely show stability. If the floor has been reached, further OCT scans may be of limited utility.
5. Has there been change with time? Figure 26.14 shows a colour-coded progression layout available with the Zeiss Cirrus OCT machine. Red shading demarcates that there is likely loss, while orange indicates possible loss.

The interpretation of disc OCTs is not as "structural" as macular OCTs, rather they are used as one piece in an overall clinical puzzle and require you to cross-correlate OCT

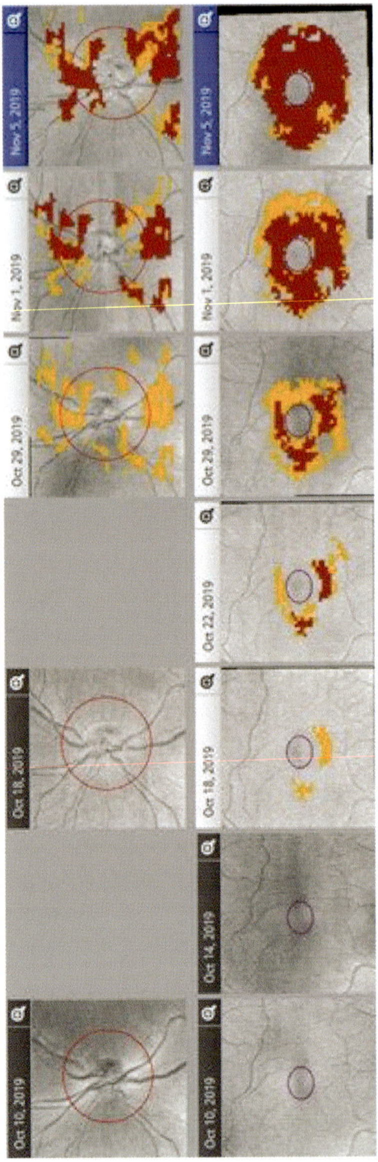

Fig. 26.14 Zeiss macular ganglion cell progression display. There is evidence of worsening peripapillary retinal nerve fibre layer thinning and macular ganglion cell loss.

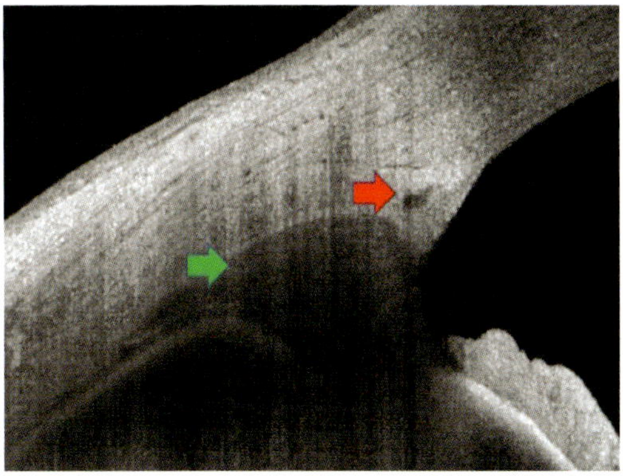

Fig. 26.15 Limited view of ciliary body (green arrow). Schlemm's canal can also be seen here (red arrow).

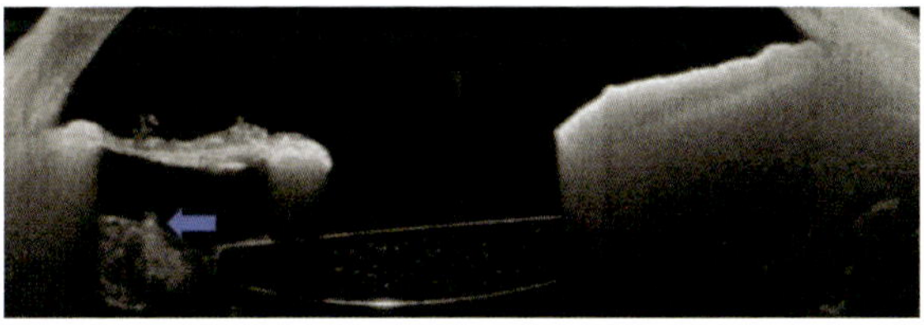

Fig. 26.16 This patient has an iris defect on the left-hand side of the scan, which allows light to pass so the ciliary body can be visualised. The small dot on top of it is a haptic from a sulcus intraocular lens (arrow). However, on the right-hand side you can see that no detail of the ciliary body is possible due to the overlying iris.

findings with any evidence of functional decline, e.g. visual field deficits.

INTERPRETATION OF IMAGES: ANTERIOR SEGMENT OCT

This is not as commonly used as disc and macular OCT. However, it is gaining popularity as an objective way of recording baseline anterior chamber angle and depth. It can also be useful in cornea clinics, for example in checking endothelial graft attachment and quantifying corneal thickness. Additionally, OCT imaging of conjunctival lesions and glaucoma surgery is gaining popularity, though the interpretation of these images is more of a sub-specialist area.

Not all OCTs can perform an anterior segment image by default, some require an additional piece of hardware that is physically attached to the front of the OCT machine. Therefore, you should check with your unit whether anterior segment OCT is available.

As OCT is an optical technique, its ability to view the ciliary body is limited due to the iris acting as a barrier to the incoming light. However, you can see that with lateral gaze, some imaging of the ciliary body is achievable, though visualisation of the ciliary processes is limited. If imaging of the ciliary body is required, a UBM (ultrasound biomicroscopy) is the best option.

INTERPRETATION OF IMAGES: OCT ANGIOGRAPHY (OCTA)

One of the most recent developments in OCT is OCTA having become available in 2014. It works through measuring the differences in light reflected when the same area is scanned at different times, the difference in reflected light equating to flow of blood through the region being scanned. This allows the flow of blood through the small vessels in the retina to be imaged and is particularly useful for looking at areas of ischaemia and capillary dropout.

However, there are limitations insofar as the scan takes longer to perform, is more sensitive to motion artefact than standard angiography, can have segmentation artefacts and in particular can suffer from projection artefacts. Projection artefacts result in superficial vessels appearing to be present in the outer retina, due to light arriving at the RPE being influenced by prior reflection from the superficial vascular plexus.

Approach to Interpreting OCTA Printouts[1]

1. **Check grid size is correct** for the purpose you need. For neovascular membrane detection small grids are fine, but for examining diabetic ischaemia larger grids are needed.
2. **Examine the en face image**: Is the foveal avascular zone in the superficial capillary plexus the right size and regularity? Are microaneurysms present? The three important en face scans are shown as the lower three images in Figure 26.17. In the superficial vascular complexes, signs of ischaemia pertaining to diabetic retinopathy may be evident. In the avascular and choroidal complexes, neovascular membranes will show as bright white vessel networks.
3. **Check segmentation lines**: These are the red lines shown in Figure 26.17 and indicate that the scan has been divided up between the different complexes correctly.

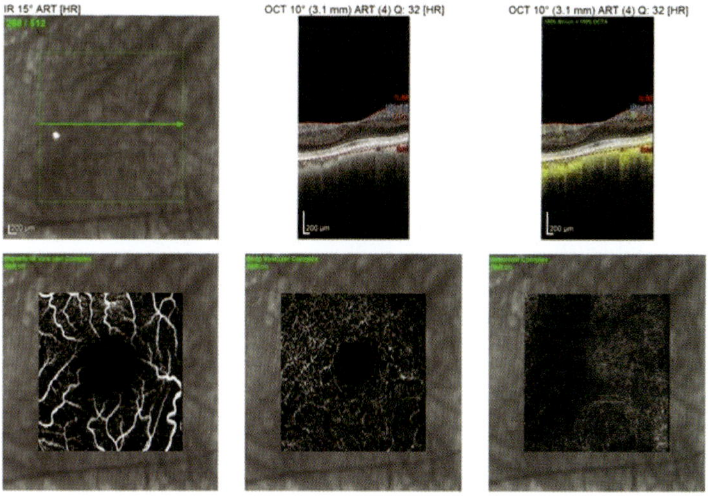

Fig. 26.17 OCTA report, the superficial vascular complex en face image shows vessels from the internal limiting membrane through to the inner plexiform layer. The deep vascular complex is from the inner nuclear layer to the outer plexiform layer. The avascular complex is from the outer plexiform layer to the outer nuclear layer. The projection of some of the superficial vessels can still faintly be seen.

4. **Compare findings en face with the transverse B scan.** Looking at just the en face view may lead to incorrect diagnosis of capillary dropout or neovascular complexes, when there may simply be vessels crossing or overlying pathology that has a masking effect, detectable from an alternative view.

CONCLUSIONS

- OCT is a widely used investigation and it is essential to be familiar with the relevant macular anatomy.
- Disc OCT is widely used. However, be mindful that it is often used as one part of a puzzle in glaucoma/neuro-ophthalmic diagnosis and monitoring. There are limitations to its use in certain eyes.
- Anterior segment OCT is useful. However, less widely used, it is still establishing a role in glaucoma and anterior segment subspecialties.

Reference

1. Greig EC, Duker JS, Waheed NK. (2020) A practical guide to optical coherence tomography angiography interpretation. *Int J Retina Vitreous* **6**(1): 55.

27

ANGIOGRAPHY

Thomas Sherman

Most units have the facility for fluorescein angiography. Indocyanine green angiography is a less universally available investigation but is common enough to need to know the interpretation of. Both investigations are generally vetted by medical retina specialists and are worth discussing with a specialist in this area or a consultant before requesting. The investigations do take a fair amount of time to perform. They also carry very small risks of significant problems like anaphylaxis from fluorescein.

FLUORESCEIN ANGIOGRAPHY

Main Indications

- To look for choroidal neovascularisation
- To assess level of ischaemia in the retina
- To detect inflammation of retinal vessels or disc
- To detect subtle neovascularisation

Practical Aspects of Fluorescein Angiography

It is good practice for patients to give formal written consent for fluorescein angiography. The purpose of the investigation is usually to provide images for diagnostic benefit.

The risks are: failure to obtain adequate quality images, nausea/vomiting, flushing, anaphylaxis to fluorescein. It is important to mention that patients will notice a discoloration of their urine temporarily.

A cannula of any gauge is needed for the procedure and usually 5 mL of 10% fluorescein is given as an IV bolus. There is usually a nurse or practitioner available to deal with cannulation and administration. However, it is useful to know how the procedure works yourself. A test dose of fluorescein (5 mL of saline with a couple of drops of fluorescein) is worth giving before the bolus to ensure no adverse reaction.

There is only sufficient time for one eye to have early phase photos/videos taken, so one eye needs to be decided as the primary eye for investigation.

Cautions

Pregnancy

There are no detailed studies on safety of fluorescein angiography in pregnant and breastfeeding mothers. If fundus fluorescein angiogram (FFA) can be avoided until post-pregnancy, this is probably the best option, and a "pump and dump" strategy for breastfeeding mothers post-FFA is probably the safest approach.

Renal Failure

Fluorescein is not known to be nephrotoxic.[1] However, it is eliminated through renal excretion so may be retained in bloodstream for longer in patients with a lower eGFR, so their urine may be fluorescent for longer.

Children

FFA can be performed in children. The main issue here is the cannulation and requiring a child to co-operate with the repeated imaging. It is possible to administer fluorescein orally. However, it will stain the teeth and oral mucosa. Though this is temporary, it can be easily mitigated by drinking the fluorescein through a straw. Usually, the fluorescein is added to orange juice to make it more appealing. The problem with oral administration is that the administration of the drug to time appearing in the retinal circulation is unpredictable and may not be to the same concentration as IV doses.

Stages of Fluorescein Angiography

From injection of fluorescein intravenously there should be a fairly rapid filling of the arterial circulation (by 12 seconds). A delay in the arm-retina time may indicate systemic atherosclerotic disease or cannulation problems.

- 10 seconds — Choroidal flush
  - This appears as a dull glow of the choroidal vasculature, masked by the overlying retinal pigment epithelium (RPE)
  - Cilioretinal artery will fill at this stage if one is present
- 12 seconds — Retinal arterial stage
  - The arteries appear bright white
- 14–15 seconds — Arteriovenous phase (aka lamellar or early venous phase)

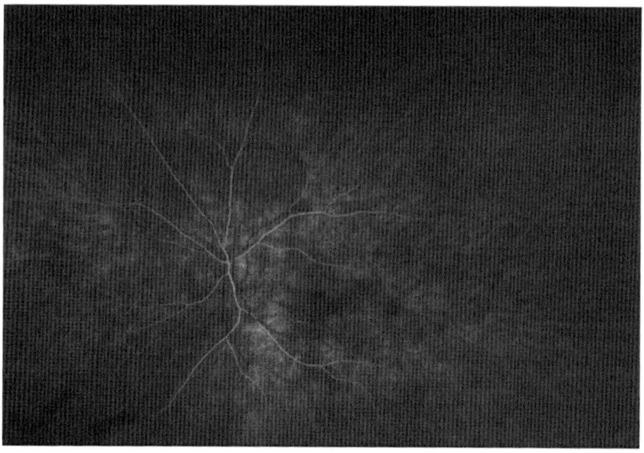

Fig. 27.1 Arterial stage.

  - Veins start to fill; the laminar flow of fluorescein through the vessels may show as hyperfluorescent columns within the veins
- 16 seconds — Venous stage
  - Veins are completely full
- Up to 30 seconds — Late venous stage
- 5–15 minutes — Late phase
  - There may be only late leakage for some choroidal neovascular membranes

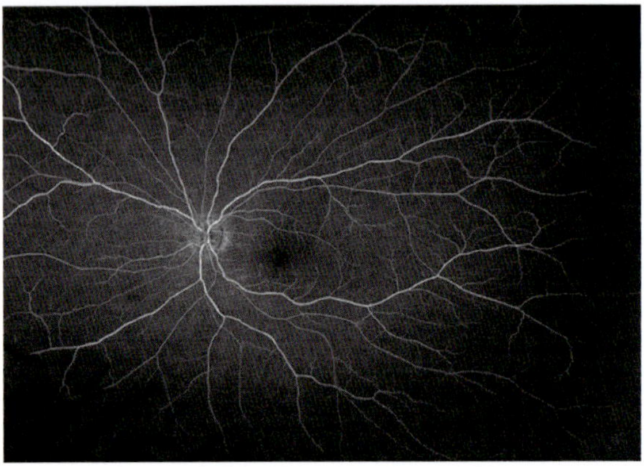

Fig. 27.2 Arteriovenous phase.

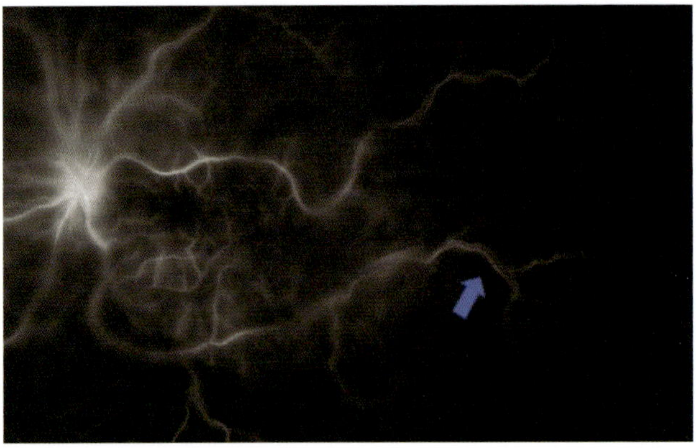

Fig. 27.3 Laminar flow seen peripherally in arteriovenous phase.

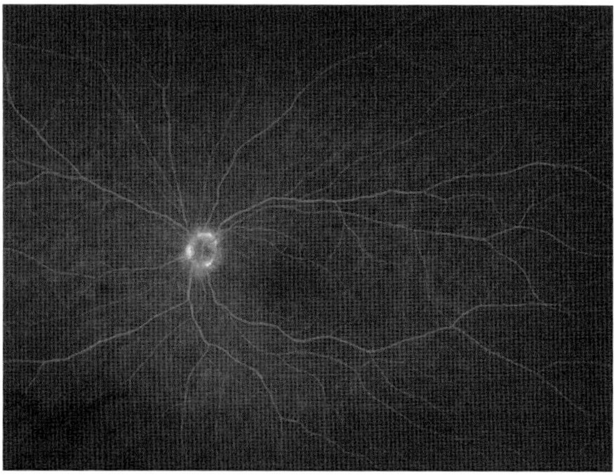

Fig. 27.4 Venous phase.

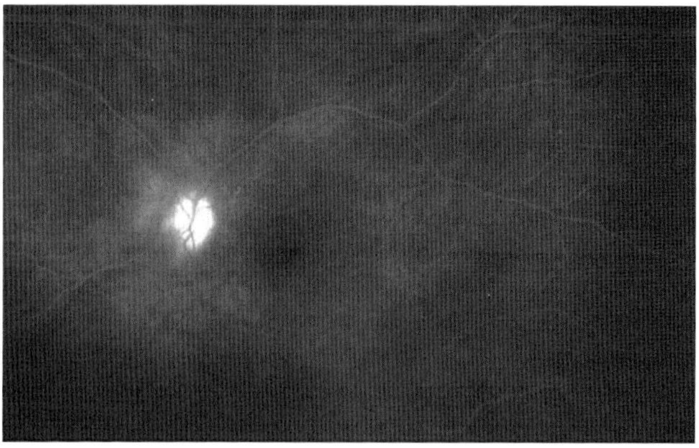

Fig. 27.5 Late phase.

Describing Findings

Hyper/hypofluorescence is a general term that describes a bright or dark appearance of the angiogram. It is either early (appearing before the venous phase) or late (appearing after venous phase). This description does not imply any process, e.g. leakage or blocking, so is an appropriate term to use when initially describing the angiogram.

Hyperfluorescence

Leakage — Not everything hyperfluorescent is "leakage". Hyperfluorescence that is seen and then expands as the angiogram progresses is leakage. This is why it is best to initially use generic terms "early hyperfluorescence" when initially asked "what does this angiogram show" and then as the angiogram progresses you can confidently state "there is leakage".

Staining — This is hyperfluorescence that does not progress in size as the angiogram continues, or diminish in intensity. It most typically indicates retinal fibrosis with disciform scars.

Window defect — This is a hyperfluorescent area that appears early and remains the same size throughout the angiogram. It is due to RPE loss leading to increased choroidal visibility.

Pooling — A hyperfluorescent area at the early phases that gradually fills.

Particular "Characteristic" Hyperfluorescent Patterns

Stippled — When describing a stippled pattern of fluorescence, this usually indicates that you are suspecting an occult CNV.

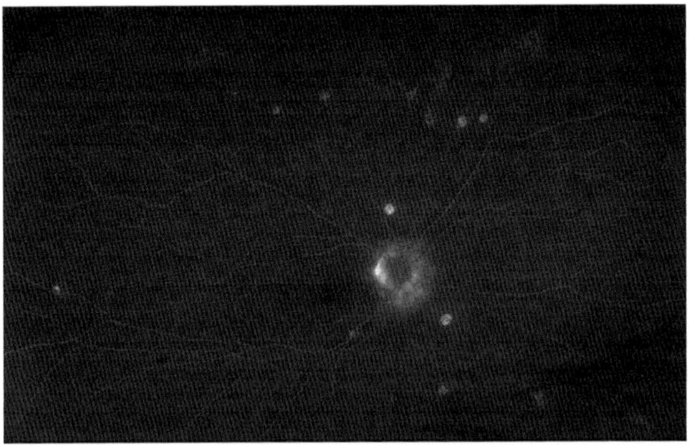

Fig. 27.6 Example of window defects as the small hyperfluorescent areas around the arcades.

Ink blot/smoke stack — This is seen in central serous retinopathy as an early hyperfluorescent dot, which then diffuses upwards before then diffusing in a horizontal direction, like smoke drifting upwards from a campfire.

Petaloid leakage — This describes a pattern of leakage seen in cystoid macular oedema which resembles flower petals around the macula.

Hypofluorescence

Blocking — This typically occurs where there is overlying preretinal haemorrhage that blocks the transmission of light from the underlying retinal vasculature. These kinds of haemorrhages can make FFAs in central retinal vein occlusions difficult to interpret in particular.

Filling defect — This is due to shutdown of the arterial vasculature, so the affected area has no dye running through it.

Foveal avascular zone — This is usually hypofluorescent in normal people. However, commenting of whether it is enlarged/irregular is of relevance when looking at how ischaemic a person's diabetic retinopathy/maculopathy is. It is usually 0.5 mm in diameter.

INDOCYANINE GREEN (ICG) ANGIOGRAPHY

Indications

- To detect polypoidal choroidal vasculopathy (an aggressive type of wet AMD)
- To assess choroidal circulation in central serous retinopathy
- Suspected choroidal inflammatory disease

Cautions

Pregnancy/breastfeeding — ICG is not believed to cross the placenta and so is deemed safe in pregnancy. However, ideally if an alternative investigation offers a means of diagnosing without administering systemic medication, this is preferred.

Practical Aspects of ICG Angiography

0.3 mg/kg of Verdye is usually given. Again this can be given through any gauge cannula and it is good practice to obtain consent and give a test dose first. Risks and benefits are the same as fluorescein angiography.

Phases

- <1 minute — Early phase, choroidal vessels full
- 3–15 minutes — Middle phase, fading of choroidal veins

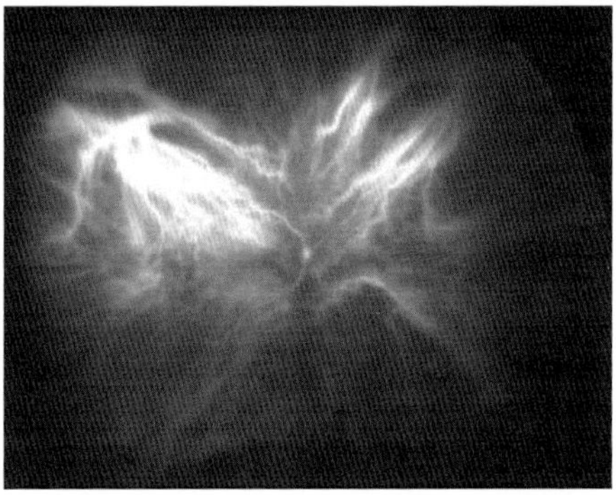

Fig. 27.7 Early phase: full choroidal vessels full of dye.

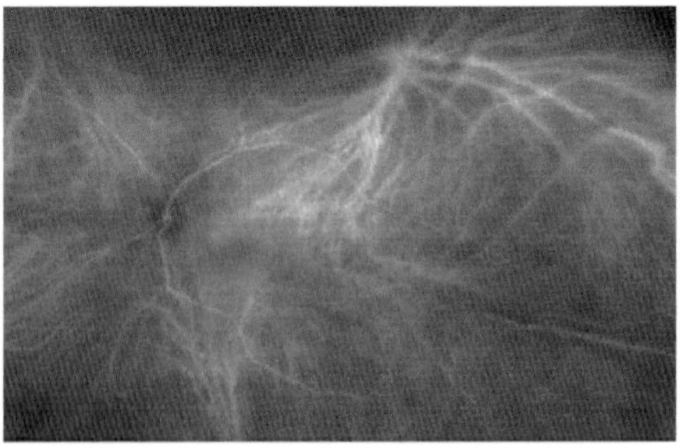

Fig. 27.8 Middle phase: the vessels have begun to fade.

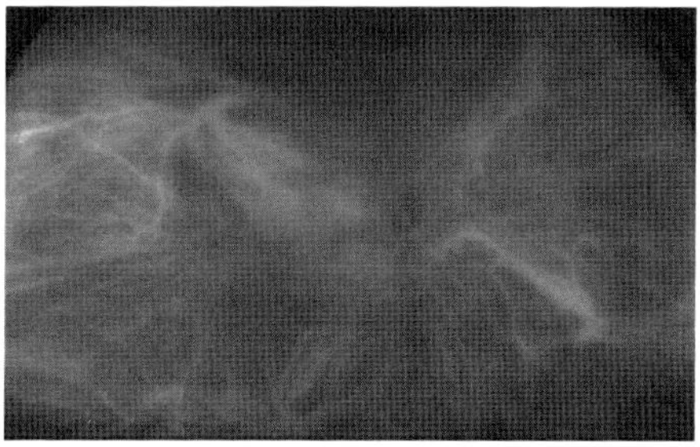

Fig. 27.9 Late phase: the choroidal vessels are becoming more hypocyanescent.

- > 15 minutes — Late phase, choroidal vasculature has a hypofluorescent appearance

Terminology

Hypercyanescence — Bright appearance on ICG that can be due to:

- RPE loss (window defect)
- Leakage
  - Hot spot — Smaller than a disc diameter and suggests PCV
  - Plaques — Areas of hypercyanescence larger than a disc diameter

Hypocyanescence — Dark appearance due to:

- Blockage — Overlying retinal haemorrhage
- Filling defect — Due to impaired choroidal circulation

OPTICAL COHERENCE TOMOGRAPHY (OCT) ANGIOGRAPHY (OCTA)

OCTA utilises Doppler shift to deduce the flow of blood through retinal capillaries and to detect areas of abnormally high or low vascularity.

OCTA does overlap with FFA in some of the questions it can answer, particularly for quantifying degrees of ischaemia. However, as there is no injected dye as part of OCTA, it lacks the ability to demonstrate leakage that can be observed in FFA. This is a very useful feature for detecting evidence of blood–retina barrier breakdown.

OCTA interpretation is a step above standard OCT interpretation. Not all centres in the UK will have OCTA capabilities at the time of writing. They are becoming more widespread, so it will become more relevant to understand their interpretation. This is covered more in the OCT chapter of this book.

CONCLUSIONS

FFA and ICG represent dynamic imaging modalities for examining retinal and choroidal perfusion. Usually, requesting this imaging is done following discussion with a consultant given the time-intensive nature and relative invasiveness. Hopefully, you will now feel more comfortable describing FFAs and ICG images. With the knowledge about how to describe these images, it is useful to then spend time with the medical retina team if your unit has dedicated FFA meetings, or on a one-to-one basis, to learn more examples of pathology that can result in these imaging findings.

Reference

1. Chung B, Lee CS. (2014) Renal function following fluorescein angiography. *Invest Ophthalmol Vis Sci* **55**(13): 258.

28

FUNDUS PHOTOGRAPHS AND OTHER FUNDUS IMAGING

Thomas Sherman

Fundus photography is a useful method of objectively documenting fundus findings that remain easily accessible for review. It is possible to use modern smartphones to take fundus photographs even without adaptors, which can be useful in out of hours or remote settings.[1] In this chapter we will also review other techniques that are used to image the fundus to provide further diagnostic information.

COLOUR FUNDUS PHOTOS

Colour fundus photos are a useful way of objectively documenting fundal pathology. The best quality fundus photos are usually obtained with pupils dilated. Probably, the most common example of fundus photography is community diabetic retinal screening. In the UK this consists of two 45° fundus images taken (two-field photography) with one photo centred on the disc and one on the macula. The original ETDRS study used a 7 stereoscopic photograph montage which is commonly seen in clinical trials on diabetic retinopathy. You may come across these when reading papers on diabetic retinopathy but they are not in widespread use in routine clinical practice.

Obtaining a fundus photograph is useful when you have to discuss retinal pathology with a retinal subspecialist, as most clinicians will be able to detect haemorrhage and neovascularisation much more easily on a photograph than on an optical coherence tomography (OCT).

Ultrawidefield Imaging

Conventional fundus imaging has a limit on the range it can extend to. Posterior pole imaging has a 50° field of view, widefield imaging includes the mid-periphery and has 100° field, then ultrawidefield imaging can potentially image to the pars plana with up to 220° field.[2]

The optos widefield cameras are widely used in the UK now and provide a 200° field of view even in undilated patients. They can be used for autofluorescent imaging and fluorescein/indocyanine green angiography as shown in the angiography chapter.

The fundus image produced by the optos is a false colour image. You will notice that images have a slight green tint to them. When looking at the photographs you will frequently see lash artefacts at the bottom of the picture (Figure 28.1). These are in fact from the upper lid. However, the fundal image itself is not inverted. Another artefact of these ultrawidefield images is that the periphery of the image is distorted, as an elliptical mirror is used to acquire the images, so structures in the periphery can look larger than they are in reality.

Some units use optos for all retinal photography. However, in units where there is both a standard field and ultrawidefield device, standard photos are useful for disc and macula imaging as they can show more detail in these structures. However, for detecting peripheral problems such as neovascularisation, retinal tears/detachments and peripheral inflammatory lesions in uveitis, ultrawidefield imaging is better. Do bear in mind that given the artefacts of peripheral distortion and eyelashes, optos

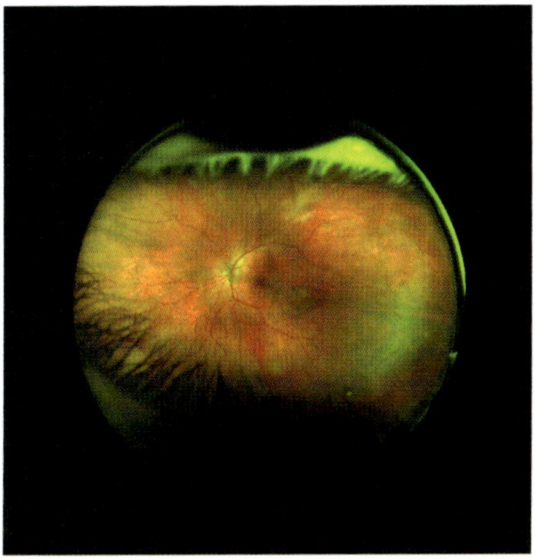

Fig. 28.1 Optos colour fundus image. Note the lash artefact at the bottom of the screen and the green tint to the periphery.

is not a substitute for a thorough peripheral retinal examination with indentation of the sclera or use of a 3-mirror lens. Relying solely on an optos image to rule out retinal tears risks missing pathology.

Monochromatic Images

Fundus images are composed of red green blue channels, like most standard photography. These channels can be separated to become monochromatic images. Different layers of the retina will reflect light in different ways, so differing structures become visible with a blue, red and green filter:

- Red filter: Retinal vessels are less visible with this filter and the choroidal detail is more visible, naevi can show up well with this filter (Figure 28.2).
- Green filter (AKA red free): The filter causes red objects to appear black, so can enhance the visibility of small bleeds and retinal vessels.
- Blue filter: Anterior retinal, e.g. retinal nerve fibre layer is best demonstrated with this filter. However, it is susceptible to large amounts of scatter.

Near-infrared reflectance image: Most modern OCT machines have a near-infrared fundus picture displayed next to the OCT (Figure 28.3). This can have similar utility to a red-free fundus image in that blood and other red structures tend to show up well on this scan.

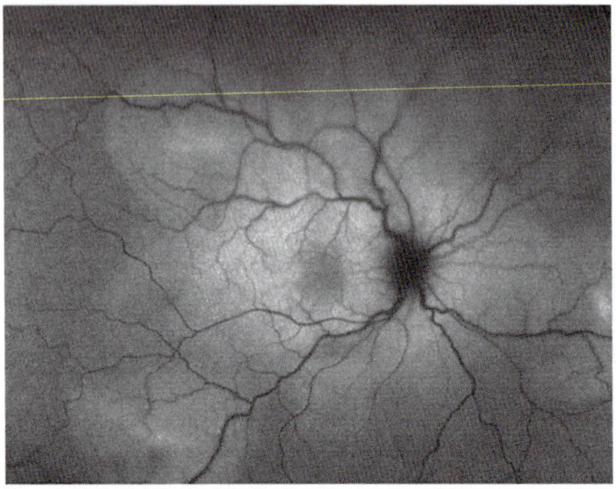

Fig. 28.2 Example red-free image showing black retinal vessels and multiple shallow choroidal effusions.

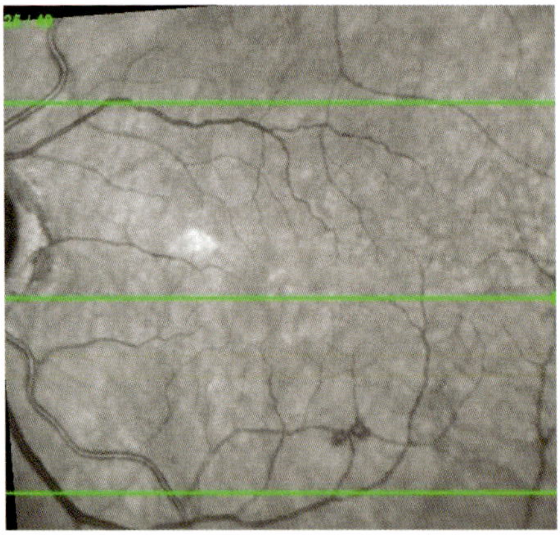

Fig. 28.3 Near-infrared image showing dark vascular arcades. Note the microaneurysm seen in the inferior arcade.

AUTOFLUORESCENCE

The retinal pigment epithelium (RPE) contains lipofuscin, a waste product that accumulates in lysosomes from vitamin A metabolism. Within lipofuscin is a substance known as A2E, which is excited by light between 430 nm and 450 nm and emits light at 560–575 nm.[3] This is the predominant structure that generates an autofluorescent signal with clinical autofluorescent imaging. Autofluorescence can provide information about RPE health. Where the RPE is accumulating lipofuscin as a result of disturbed metabolism, increased autofluorescence is seen. Where RPE has died, it will be visualised as hypoautofluorescent. Autofluorescence can be particularly useful in looking for subtle retinal pathology, such as the case in Figure 28.4.

Autofluorescence images can be obtained by blue light or green light autofluorescence. Each produces slightly different images. An example of a blue light autofluorescence imaging system is the Heidelberg Spectralis® (488 nm). The optos widefield camera uses a green light autofluorescence (532 nm).[4] Both of these machines are confocal scanning laser ophthalmoscopes. They use a modified pinhole system to capture light

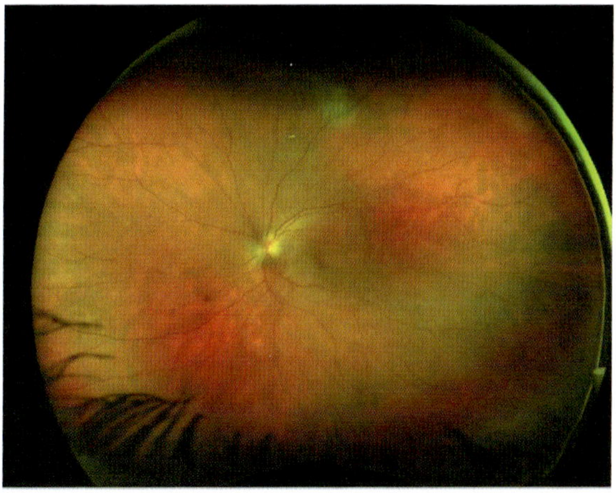

Fig. 28.4A Subtle perimacular pathology visible on an optos fundus photograph.

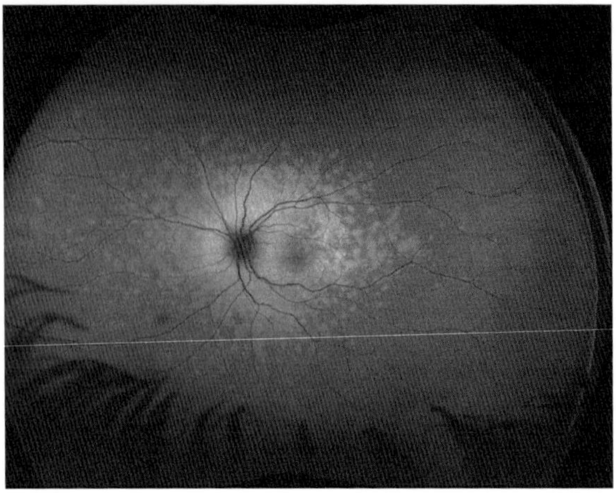

Fig. 28.4B Autofluorescent image of the same retina as Figure 28.4A. There are widespread areas of hyperautofluorescence around the disc.

only from the excited retinal structures, eliminating scattered light from other structures such as the lens to produce a clear image. Fundus cameras do not use this system but can still be used to generate autofluorescent images. These cameras include the Zeiss Visucam and Topcon TRC-50DX both of which use blue light autofluorescence. The best images for autofluorescence imaging are usually obtained with dilated pupils.

Indications for autofluorescent imaging include suspicion of any condition where the health of the RPE is felt to be compromised. One of the most common indications is for the detection of hydroxychloroquine maculopathy. Here, in the early stages, a paracentral hyperautofluorescent ring around the macula is seen, before then becoming hypoautofluorescent in advanced disease. These features may not be visible on slit-lamp examination of the macula or even OCT.

Other retinal problems which autofluorescence is useful for examining are the white dot syndromes. Where photoreceptor loss occurs, the underlying RPE becomes unmasked and therefore hyperautofluorescence results, as Figure 28.5 shows. In one type of white dot syndrome, punctate inner choroidopathy (PIC), active lesions can be seen as hyperautofluorescent rings

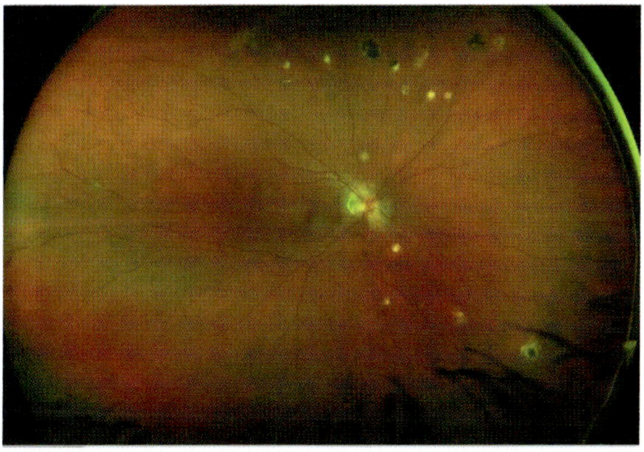

Fig. 28.5A The fellow eye shows some old chorioretinal scars which show up black on autofluorescence due to their lack of fluorophores.

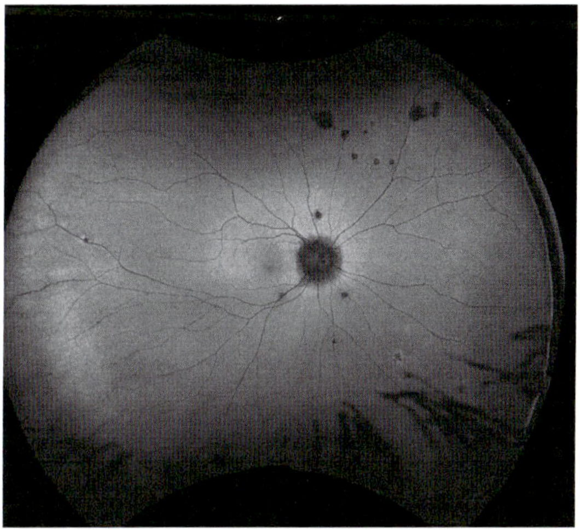

Fig. 28.5B Autofluorescence of retinal scars.

surrounding a hypoautofluorescent centre. This is due to loss of the RPE as the inflammatory sub-RPE nodule breaks through, with surrounding photoreceptor loss that causes hyperautofluorescence.

Finally, autofluorescence of the optic nerve head can be performed to look for optic disc drusen. However, these drusen

Table 28.1 Causes of Hypoautofluorescence.

	Reduced RPE lipofuscin	Blockage from material anterior to RPE
Example	RPE atrophy RPE tear	Opaque media Normal macular pigment Retinal haemorrhages Fibrosis/scarring

Adapted from Yung *et al.*[5]

Table 28.2 Causes of Hyperautofluorescence.

	Increased lipofuscin in RPE	Subretinal autofluorescent material	Window defect (loss of photoreceptors)	Other autofluorescent material
Example	Stargardt's disease Pattern dystrophies	Vitelliform Central serous chorioretinopathy (CSR)	White dot syndrome Macular telangiectasia type II CSR	Optic disc drusen Astrocytic hamartoma

Adapted from Yung *et al.*[5]

need to be fairly superficial to produce a hyperautofluorescent signal. Deeper buried drusen will not be visible on autofluorescence. Tables 28.1 and 28.2 include the causes of low or high autofluorescent levels and also detail some of the causes of these.

This patient's colour widefield image (Figure 28.4) may look normal at first (there are actually subtle flec-like areas around the macula). However, the autofluorescence image shows dramatic evidence of disturbed RPE function. This patient was diagnosed with multiple evanescent white dot syndrome (MEWDS), a type of rare inflammatory chorioretinopathy.

CONCLUSIONS

Fundus photography is a relatively straightforward investigation but is particularly useful for documentation purposes.

Autofluorescence is a very useful form of fundal imaging for assessing RPE health and has particular importance in hydroxychloroquine screening, the investigation of inflammatory chorioretinal disease and inherited retinal dystrophies.

References

1. Anon. Smartphone Funduscopy — How to Use Smartphone to Take Fundus Photographs — EyeWiki. Available at: https://eyewiki.aao.org/Smartphone_Funduscopy_-_How_to_Use_Smartphone_to_Take_Fundus_Photographs [Accessed October 17, 2021].
2. Patel SN, Shi A, Wibbelsman TD, Klufas MA. (2020) Ultra-widefield retinal imaging: an update on recent advances. *Ther Adv Ophthalmol* **12**: 2515841419899495.
3. Delori FC, Goger DG, Dorey CK. (2001) Age-related accumulation and spatial distribution of lipofuscin in RPE of normal subjects. *Invest Ophthalmol Vis Sci* **42**(8): 1855–1866.
4. Bittencourt MG, Hassan M, Halim MS, *et al.* (2019) Blue light versus green light fundus autofluorescence in normal subjects and in patients with retinochoroidopathy secondary to retinal and uveitic diseases. *J Ophthalmic Inflamm Infect* **9**: 1.
5. Yung M, Klufas MA, Sarraf D. (2016) Clinical applications of fundus autofluorescence in retinal disease. *Int J Retina Vitreous* **2**(1): 12.

29

VISUAL FIELD TESTING

Thomas Sherman

Visual field testing is an important, subjective test of patients' central and peripheral vision sensitivity to light stimuli. It is most commonly applied in glaucoma clinics and neuro-ophthalmic clinics. However, its application can extend to any situation where one wants to create a spatial map of sensitivity across a subject's visual field. In a separate book (Fundamentals of Glaucoma, World Scientific), we have written about visual field testing in glaucoma. Here we provide an overview of field testing outside of glaucoma applications specifically.

CONFRONTATIONAL TESTING

Outside of ophthalmology, confrontational visual field testing is the mainstay of visual field examination. Often this involves presenting a finger or coloured pin into the visual field to obtain a crude map of the patient's peripheral vision. This can be done in such a way to make it a useful assessment of the peripheral vision. It is sensitive enough to map out quadrantanopias and hemianopias, and enlargement of the blind spot can be clinically detectable with careful positioning of the patient.

CONFRONTATIONAL FIELDS: EXAMINATION

Ensure that you are sat straight in front of the patient at the same level. There should be about a metre distance between you.

Binocular Field Screen

The patient has both eyes open and examiner has both hands held up shoulder's width apart.

"Point to the hand you see moving", move one hand, then the other, then both.

Result: A patient with a left homonymous hemianopia will fail to detect the left hand moving with a sufficiently dense field defect (beware that some hemianopias may not occupy the full extent of the hemifield and may not be dense to the extent that your hand cannot be detected).

Monocular Field Screen

"Please cover one eye with your hand and look straight ahead at me. Can you see all of my face? Are any parts missing".

Result: Sufficiently dense scotomas may be detected in this way as missing facial features. Bitemporal defects may manifest themselves as the inability to detect the lateral peripheries.

Quadrant Screen

"Cover one eye; look at my eye; tell me how many fingers you see (alternate between one and two fingers displayed in each quadrant".

You can then draw a 2 × 2 grid with "CF" in each segment that this was seen in for documentation.

Confrontational Field Testing: Author's Opinion

Confrontational field testing in settings where access to visual fields is not possible, out of hours or on call for example, is useful. However, it has nowhere near the ability to detect the sensitivity of the visual field in the way that automated visual field testing can. It cannot be reliably mapped and followed up so really retains utility as a gross screening exam. However, occasionally you will encounter patients whose automated visual field test shows widespread dense defects that may be of questionable reliability. In these settings, it is useful to do a confrontational test to confirm if the extent of these defects really represents a genuine loss of visual field rather than a cognitive difficulty in performing automated visual field tests.

QUANTIFYING THE VISUAL FIELD

A normal visual field extends approximately 90° temporally, 60° nasally, 60° superiorly and 70° inferiorly. It has a different range of sensitivity across it, with the central field being most sensitive. In the periphery, sensitivity declines and at the optic nerve is the blind spot. This creates the overall "hill of vision" shown in Figure 29.1.

The earliest form of field tests involved using a black tangent screen with a target printed onto it. A black wand held by a perimetrist wearing a long black glove would then be placed on the screen and a map could be made of the visual field if the patient's distance from the screen was kept constant. This had the advan-

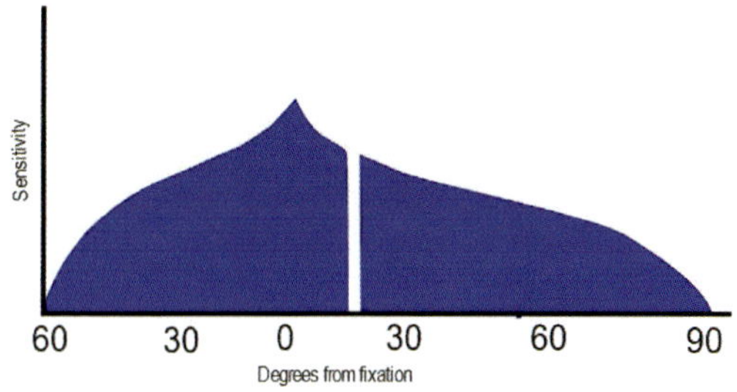

Fig. 29.1 Hill of vision showing maximum sensitivity at the fovea with a drop off peripherally and a blind spot at around 15° temporally. Average height is approximately 6°–9° and width is 5°–6° depending on target size.[1] The left-hand side of the graph is nasal and the right temporal in direction.

tage of having a perimetrist constantly assessing the patient's attention and doing the test at their pace. However, it is time consuming and insensitive to small changes. Tangent screen testing does not tend to be performed in the UK anymore. However, it does still have a role in less economically developed areas.

Goldmann Visual Field Testing

Goldmann field testing uses a "goldfish bowl" (Figure 29.2) style machine with a set level of background illumination and a manually operated arm with a variable intensity/size light stimulus on one end and a connection to a pen on the other. A piece of paper with field markings is slotted to the back of the machine and the field is manually drawn with different isoptres represent-

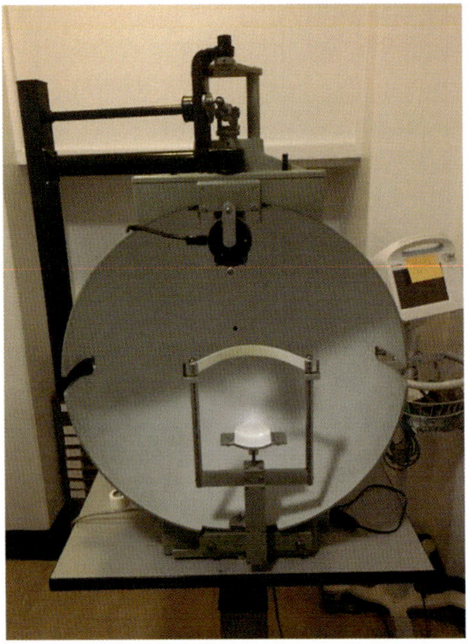

Fig. 29.2 Goldmann visual field machine, the patient places their chin on the chinrest. The perimetrist is sat behind the bowl and fixation can be observed through a hole in the bowl. The black arm swings inwards with a fixation light, adjusting in size and intensity by the perimetrist. When the patient first sees it, they press a buzzer and the position is recorded on a sheet.

ing the different intensity stimuli and the extent to which they are seen.

This test is more time consuming than automated field testing. It can take around 45 minutes to test both eyes depending on the patient and perimetrist. However, it is often considered the 'gold standard' neuro-ophthalmic visual field. Some patients simply cannot perform an accurate Humphrey visual field (HVF), so are often referred for Goldmann visual fields to accurately ascertain the level of field impairment.

Figure 29.3 shows an example Goldmann visual field from a patient with papilloedema. You can see that several isoptres are drawn and their extent can be read off the chart markings in degrees from fixation. The blind spot is specifically mapped out. In this case, it is enlarged. The colour code for the different size and intensity stimuli are detailed in the lower right-hand box. There is no set colour coding so this must be marked to make it clear which isoptres correspond to which stimulus. The stimuli go from I to V in roman numerals to indicate size (V is the largest). Each numeral upwards is a change by a factor

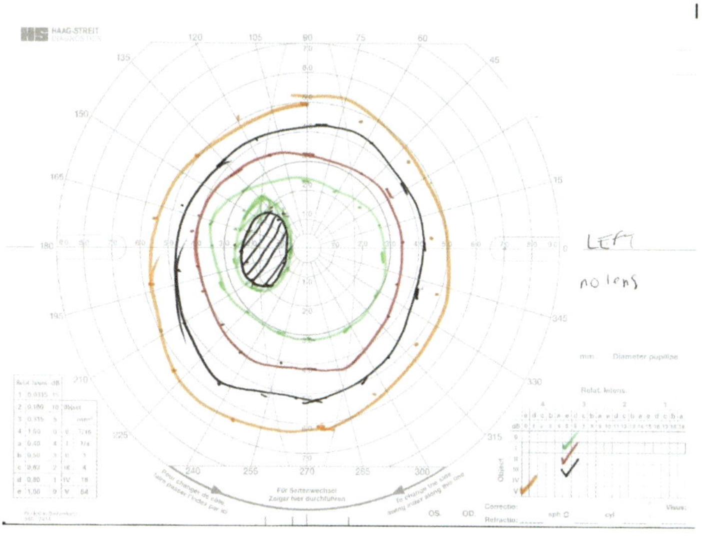

Fig. 29.3 Goldmann visual field showing enlarged blind spot in a patient with papilloedema.

of 2. The Arabic numeral ranges from 1 to 4 and increases brightness by 3.15 times the previous value (1 dimmest – 4 brightest). The lowercase letter indicates whether a filter was applied to titrate the luminance downwards by 0.1 log unit. The letter "a" signifies the darkest filter and "e" the lightest. Therefore, the biggest and brightest stimulus is V4e.

Patients with functional visual symptoms may also display typical patterns of Goldmann visual fields such as crossing isoptres, and spiralling field defects (Figures 29.4 and 29.5) so it can be useful for demonstrating that this condition is present.

When interpreting a Goldmann visual field you are essentially examining the extent of each isoptre and comparing this between visits. The blind spot size should also be evaluated and compared between visits.

Goldmann visual fields are limited by their application for glaucoma. Although it can be used in this setting, it lacks the same ability to define the sensitivity of each area of the visual field in the same time that an automated field test can. There is an automated Goldmann (the Octopus perimeter), which is said to have a similar reliability of Goldmann visual field testing. However, this does not have the same operator intense approach to monitoring the patient as a traditional manual Goldmann perimetry.

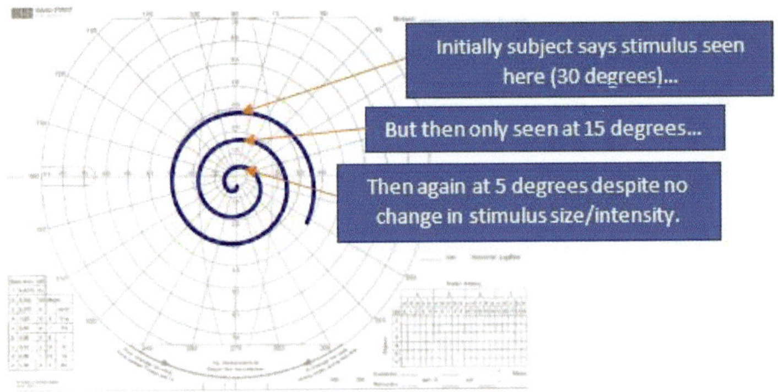

Fig. 29.4 Spiralling field. If you suspect a functional diagnosis, it is helpful to inform the perimetrist and they can specifically test for spiralling.

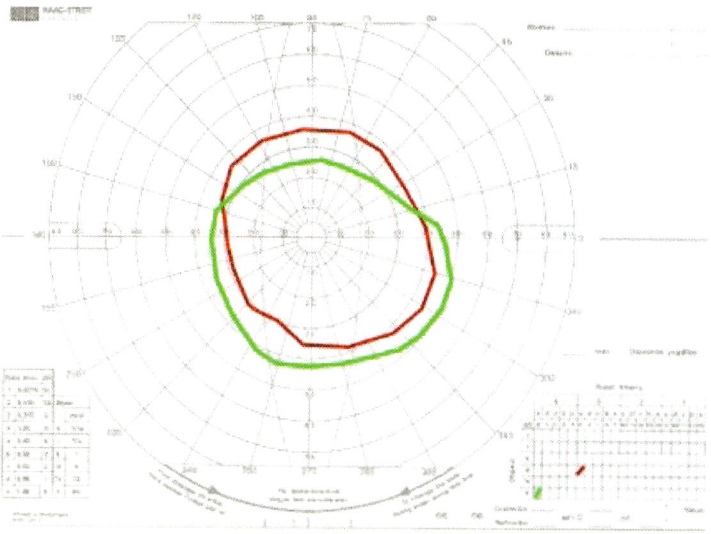

Fig. 29.5 Crossing isoptres: Here the green V stimulus is larger than the red III stimulus. At the superior aspect of the field however, the patient can see the smaller stimulus further out than the larger stimulus, so the isoptres cross. This does not make physiological sense.

Automated Visual Field Testing

This is by far the commonest form of visual field testing. There are multiple brands of visual field machines available but the most common is the HVF machine (Zeiss). The purpose of this chapter is not to provide you with detailed training in how to perform visual field testing, but to explain some of the technical aspects of doing a visual field that allow you to understand its interpretation.

How Does the Machine Work?

The HVF machine has a fixed intensity background light (31.5 apostilbs). Against this fixed luminance background, lights are shone in various positions around the visual field that vary in intensity. They are stepped up and down in their luminance and the patient clicks a handheld button each time they can see the stimulus. To ensure that the field is mapped appropriately, they must maintain fixation on an orange light in the middle of the background. A perimetrist should be watching the patient whilst they do the test to ensure that fixation is being maintained and that the patient is always in the correct position for the test.

Visual Field Testing Types

The 24-2 test is the most commonly used test that is principally for use in glaucoma. For neuro-ophthalmic investigation, a 30-2 test is usually selected. The 24- and 30-2 are so named because they test 24 or 30 degrees from fixation and are the second iteration of a testing strategy that has been adapted so that points are tested either side of the vertical and horizontal midline. The 10-2 test is designed to focus on the central vision and is used in hydroxycholorquine testing and to quantify defects from macular disease.

There are other patterns contained within the HVF machine that are seldom used, for example the 60-4 test that tests from 30° to 60° peripherally. Additionally, there is the relatively new 24-2C, which tests 10 additional points from the central 10° to provide more information about the central field than a standard 24-2.[2] The normal 24-2 test only includes 12 points tested in the central 10° field, whereas the 10-2 tests 68 points in the same area (Table 29.1)!

Testing Strategies

The Swedish Interactive Thresholding Algorithm (SITA) is the standard strategy for threshold visual field testing. It uses real-time probability estimates to determine step sizes needed when testing visual field thresholds. The SITA Standard strategy and

Table 29.1 Test Patterns for HVF.

	Number of points tested	Extent
10-2	68	Central 10° from fixation
24-2	54	Central 24° (with further points tested nasally)
30-2	76	Central 30° from fixation

the SITA fast strategy are the two main algorithms in use today. There is now a recently developed SITA faster algorithm which is said to reduce test time even further.[3] SITA standard was considered the gold standard for a long time. It is still widely used in clinical trials for glaucoma. It takes around 3–7 minutes to complete the test (per eye).

SITA fast takes around 2–5 minutes but this is not because it is a "faster" test or tests less points. Instead, it stops testing when a level of certainty has been reached about the visual field sensitivity. The SITA standard requires greater certainty before testing can be stopped. With this in mind, variability between tests can potentially increase more with SITA fast testing, as potentially patient error can be incorporated more easily than a SITA standard test. However, a balance has to be struck between ease and availability of testing versus reliability. Most centres now use SITA fast routinely in their glaucoma clinics due to the high volumes of tests needed. The new SITA faster test takes on average 3 minutes[3] to perform. It is still a rather new testing strategy so has yet to establish its place and value in routine clinical practice.

Examining the Visual Field: Assessing Reliability

Visual field testing can be quite demanding for patients to go through. It is therefore important to assess reliability parameters to make sure that the visual field test in front of you is comparable to previous ones and the conclusions drawn from it are meaningful. Several parameters help you to make this judgement:

False positives: These are registered every time the patient has acknowledged a stimulus, despite one not being presented. Where this is >15% the reliability is heavily compromised.

Fixation losses: Fixation losses occur when the patient identifies that they have seen a stimulus that the machine has mapped the blind spot to, as the position of the blind spot has moved. This is also how some visual fields can be generated with a seemingly absent blind spot. Small discs or large refractive error can sometimes result in the machine being overly sensitive to fixation losses despite patients having had good fixation during testing.

False negatives: These are generated when a patient identifies a stimulus of greater luminance at a point where they had previously registered seeing only a lower intensity stimulus. This should usually be <20%. However, individuals with advanced glaucoma may have false negatives register inappropriately high due to variability in field sensitivity, so a high level of false negatives may not necessarily invalidate a field test in the same way false positives do.

Test duration: Where tests take a long time (for example >5 minutes per eye) patient fatigue is likely to have set in or there may have had to be repeated pauses in the test, which can affect reliability. This is a rather soft index to be considered as a long test is not necessarily unreliable *per se*.

Gaze tracker: At the bottom of the field report, a gaze tracker printout is present. Where there are large spikes in this gaze trace, fixation is likely to have been suboptimal. Again, this is a soft reliability index that does not usually invalidate a test.

With any field test, it is important to correlate the results clinically. A severely depressed visual field with a normal optic nerve head may mean that there is a retrobulbar site of pathology, or it may mean that the patient was unable to cope with field testing. Just as we mentioned functional visual fields in the Goldmann section, with HVF testing a "clover leaf" pattern indicates a potential diagnosis of functional visual loss or simply low engagement with the test as mentioned in Figure 29.6.

Remember that field testing is ultimately subjective and can fluctuate. Sometimes patients must be reminded how best to perform the test. Figure 29.7 shows a patient who experienced an unexplained decline in their visual field, only to be retested with a reminder on how to take the test and achieved a dramatic improvement.

Examining the Visual Field: Report Maps (Figure 29.10)

Threshold sensitivity map (top left): These numerical values at each test point show how many decibels of attenuation (i.e. how much decrease in luminance) was achieved at each test

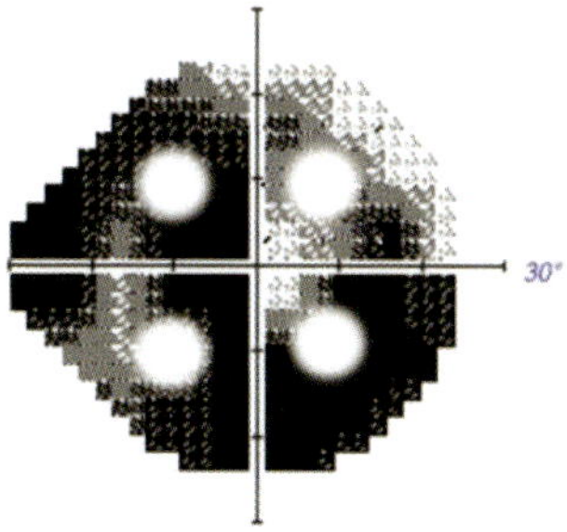

Fig. 29.6 Schematic overlay of a clover leaf appearance in a 24-2 field. The visual field stimuli are normally presented in the four areas with white circles. The patient identifies that they can see these so display white. They then lose interest in doing the rest of the test so the remaining areas appear blacked out.

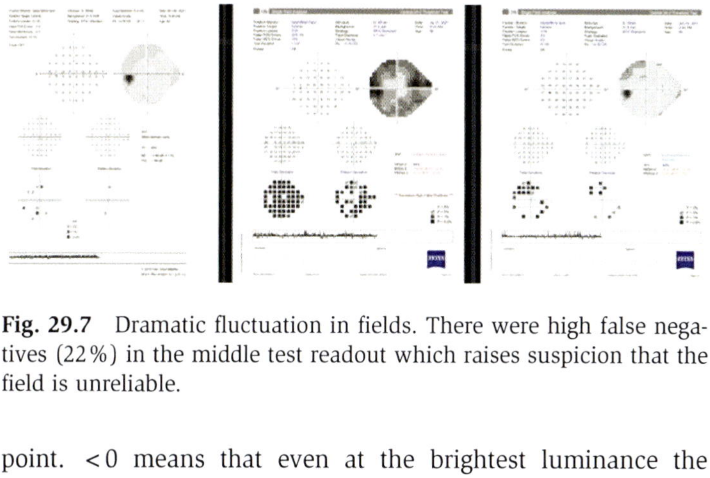

Fig. 29.7 Dramatic fluctuation in fields. There were high false negatives (22%) in the middle test readout which raises suspicion that the field is unreliable.

point. <0 means that even at the brightest luminance the stimulus was not seen, 0 means the stimulus was seen but only at the brightest intensity. Conversely, a value of 50 means that the light was maximally attenuated, which is not usually visible in normal physiological conditions. Values around 40 dB of attenuation are likely supraphysiological, suggesting false positives. These are the raw data from which other maps are plotted.

Greyscale map (top right): A graphical depiction of the threshold sensitivity map, with darker areas representing more severe areas of sensitivity loss. Although instinctively your eye is drawn to the greyscale, it is not age adjusted nor adjusted for the overall hill of vision as mentioned later.

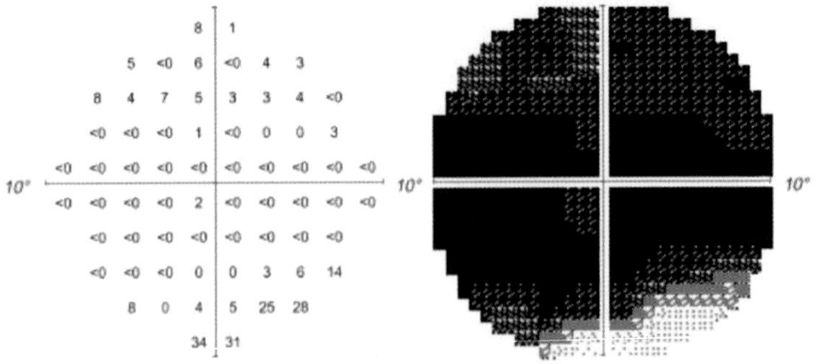

Fig. 29.8 A 10-2 field test showing severe widespread depression from advanced glaucoma. You can see how there is a preserved area of vision inferiorly where higher levels of stimulus attenuation are possible. Centrally, no stimulus attenuation was possible. You can see that from inferior towards the centre the field gradually depresses to maximum centrally. This gradual change is typical of glaucoma. In cortical disease, there is typically a sharp demarcation between normal areas and areas of maximal depression.

Total deviation map (bottom left): This shows areas of reduced sensitivity compared to an age-matched cohort, a p-value is assigned to quantify the certainty that a particular point departs from the normal sensitivity.

Pattern deviation map (bottom right): This shows areas of reduced sensitivity adjusting for the overall hill of vision. This map represents a method of adjusting for media opacities, which reduce the overall sensitivity of the visual field by reducing the amount of light entering the eye. By adjusting for this, discrete areas of reduced sensitivity (due to optic nerve disease or focal retinal disease) can be visualised. Figure 29.9 depicts this concept as a graphic.

Examining the Visual Field: Report Indices

MD (mean deviation): This is an average of the overall departure from age-adjusted normal threshold sensitivity and gives an overall figure of severity for the visual field. For glaucoma, the Hodapp–Parrish–Anderson criteria are a widely

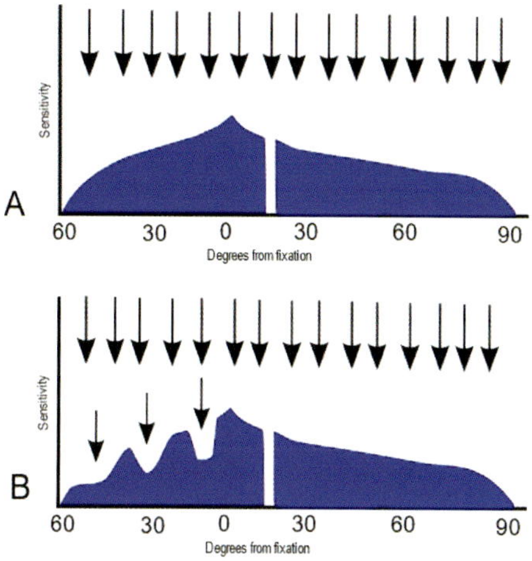

Fig. 29.9 (A) The overall hill of vision is reduced from cataract, which causes an even reduction in light entering the eye. The hill has the same shape as normal, but a visual field map will show widespread depression as the sensitivity indices are below that expected. (B) The patient has cataract and glaucoma. The cataract has caused widespread field depression, but the glaucoma has caused loss of ganglion cells selectively, resulting in a nasal field defect. Here you can see that the pattern of the hill contour has changed and there is greater variability in sensitivity across the field. This results in a higher PSD and a defect in the nasal aspect of the pattern deviation map.

used set of criteria with MD cutoffs for mild, moderate and severe glaucoma. Mild is better than −6 dB, moderate is −6 dB to −12 dB and severe worse than −12 dB. The criteria also judge glaucoma severity according to the location of the field defect in relation to fixation.

PSD (pattern standard deviation): This shows how wide the distribution of threshold sensitivities are, how "irregular" a field is. Therefore, in advanced overall field loss or perfect uniform vision, the value will be similar.

VFI (visual field index): A similar parameter to mean deviation. However, it is weighted to the central visual field. It is an index that gives an idea of the overall sensitivity of the patient's visual field expressed as a percentage.

GHT (glaucoma hemifield test): This specifically examines the differences between the superior and inferior hemifield to test for asymmetry that may suggest a diagnosis of glaucoma. It will report as either within normal limits, borderline or outside normal limits. You should not rely on it in isolation to diagnose glaucoma.

A useful way of thinking about MD and PSD is that the MD represents a numerical representation of the total deviation map, and the more negative it is, the worse the overall field is. The PSD

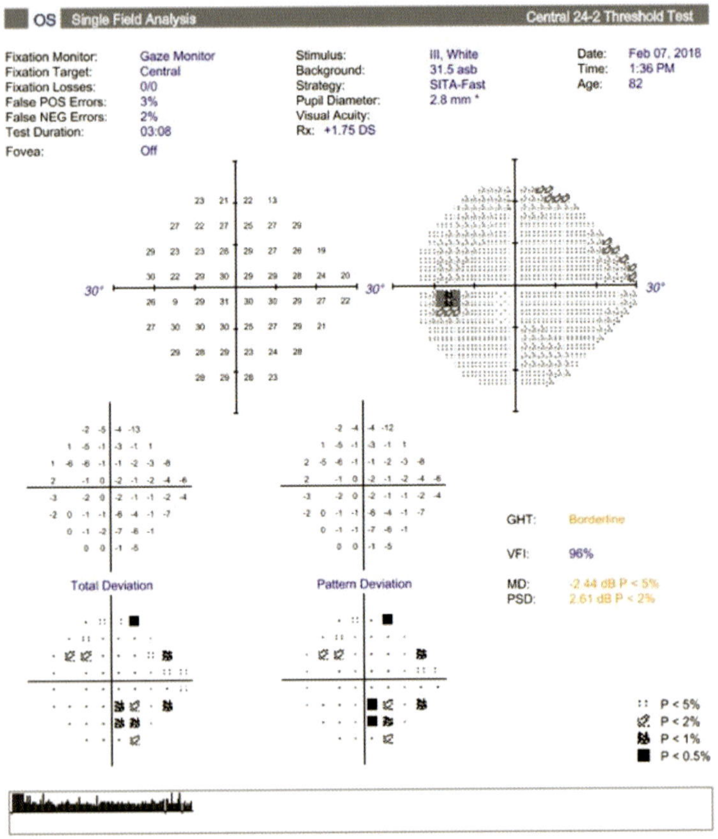

Fig. 29.10 Example 24-2 printout for a left eye with no significant field defect. A few areas show reduced sensitivity but were not clinically significant. Additionally, there is an erratic gaze trace visible at the bottom of the field.

contrasts with this in that it is a numerical representation of the pattern deviation map and a higher value means that there is much more regional variation in sensitivity. For example, in severe glaucoma with an altitudinal defect, the PSD value will be high.

Summary: Interpreting the Visual Field Report

Below is a checklist to work through which provides a general approach to interpreting the visual field readout.

1. Is this the right patient, correct date, correct testing strategy?
2. How reliable was the field:
   - What are the false positives?
   - What are the false negatives?
   - What are the fixation losses?
   - Are there any comments from the perimetrist about how the patient performed during the test?
   - What strength lens was used? (strong prescriptions can cause rim artefacts). For presbyopic patients a +3.00 lens should be added to their distance correction, for non-presbyopes their standard distance prescription is used.
   - How long did the test take?
   - Which eye was tested first?
   - Are there signs of a clover leaf pattern suggesting non-organic field defect?
   - Does this (severely depressed) field fit with a confrontational examination and the measured acuity/colour vision/pupil examination?
3. Look at greyscale to get an overall idea of the defect
4. Look at the pattern deviation to judge changes adjusted for media opacities
5. The overall MD or VFI will give an idea of "overall severity" of any field defect
6. Compare to previous fields
   - The GPA (guided progression analysis) printout is invaluable for this purpose. It will allow easy calculation of rate of dB loss and can be adjusted to remove inaccurate visual fields. Figure 29.11 shows an example.

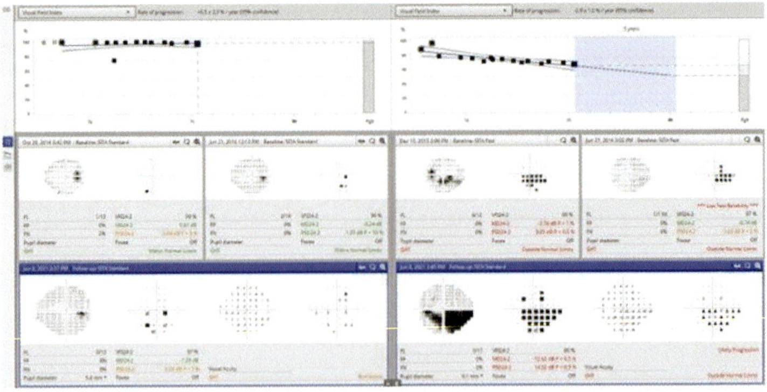

Fig. 29.11 GPA printout showing marked decline in the left eye from baseline compared to stability (flat blue trend line) in the right eye. However, bear in mind that the GPA trace can be adjusted. In this case the patient had a trabeculectomy after the third field test since then the individual fields (represented by black squares) have all been along a flat line. So here, the unadjusted GPA will overestimate the rate of progression. As there are more than five reliable fields present, the GPA can plot an estimated rate of change over the next 5 years. The bottom maps represent a probability map of individual points judged to have progressed, with black triangles indicating that >2 consecutive tests have shown progression at that point. Half triangles mean that progression has occurred at 2 consecutive tests and white triangles mean that the current test has shown statistically significant worsening in sensitivity from the previous test.

Testing for Driving Purposes

In the UK, safety to drive is ultimately decided by the DVLA. The DVLA (at the time of writing) have a contract secured with a leading high street optician to conduct all of their visual field tests for the purposes of judging fitness to drive. However, many patients naturally want to know if they are safe to drive when they come to eye clinic. If you have immediate concerns based on someone's visual field tests, it is worth advising them to not drive and speak to the DVLA about formal testing of their suitability to drive. In some cases, it may not be clear cut as to whether someone is safe to drive or not. In these cases, it is best to refer the patient to self-declare their visual field problem to the DVLA.

Esterman Visual Field Testing

The Esterman visual field test is a suprathreshold field test (i.e. instead of titrating luminance to find the threshold at which a stimulus is only just perceptible, a bright stimulus of a fixed luminance is presented). The binocular test is used for gauging fitness to drive. It extends 150° to each temporal field and tests 120 points. It can also be done as a monocular test, which tests 75° temporal and 60° nasally with 100 points in total. An example of a binocular Esterman is shown in Figure 29.12.

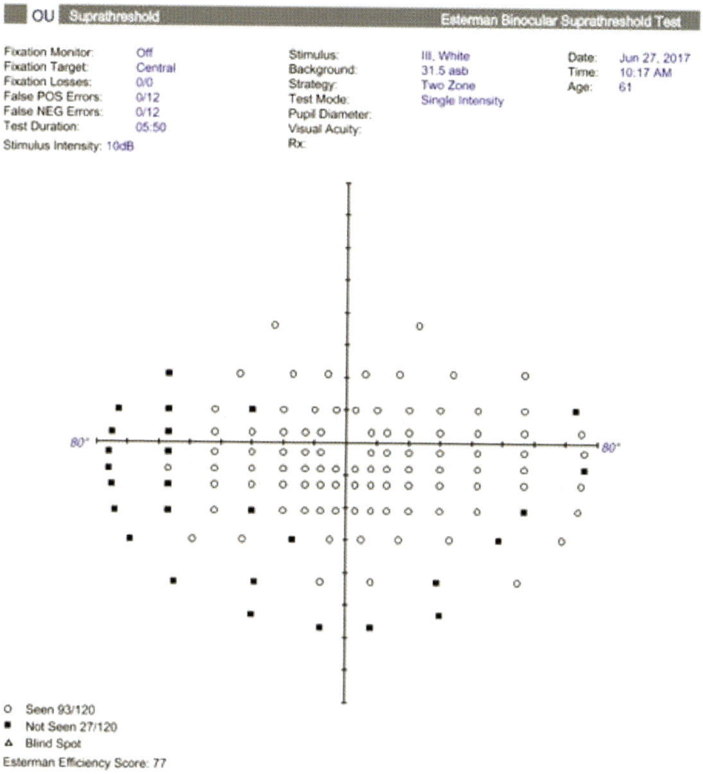

Fig. 29.12 Esterman visual field test. Note the black squares show stimuli not identified and the circles show stimuli seen. There is no plotting of visual sensitivity as this is a suprathreshold test of the visual field.

CONCLUSIONS

- Visual field testing is either confrontational, static, kinetic (manual) or kinetic (automated).
- Fields vary in reliability and there can sometimes be much at stake, e.g. invasive glaucoma surgery or even neurosurgery. It is usually better to get more data before basing the decision to operate on one field test. "Measure twice, cut once!"
- Think about the necessity of testing and whether fields are truly required, given the time it takes to perform them. Maybe your patient needs to be booked for a separate fields only appointment? Maybe only one eye should be tested per visit? Maybe it is best not to do field testing at all and use disc optical coherence tomography monitoring? It can be greatly frustrating for perimetrists and patients when people who are known to not be able to do field tests are nonetheless asked to perform them.

References

1. Cheung S-H, McHugh KM, Legge GE. (2005) Size and Location of the Physiological Blind Spot: Effects of Age and Target Size. *Invest Ophthalmol Vis Sci* **46**(13): 4784.
2. Yamane MLM, Odel JG. (2021) Introducing the 24-2C Visual Field Test in Neuro-Ophthalmology. *J Neuroophthalmol* **41**(4): e606.
3. Heijl A, Patella VM, Chong LX, *et al.* (2019) A New SITA Perimetric Threshold Testing Algorithm: Construction and a Multicenter Clinical Study. *Am J Ophthalmol* **198**: 154–165.

30

OPHTHALMIC ULTRASOUND

Thomas Sherman

Ophthalmic ultrasound is an invaluable tool for assessing the structure of the eye, especially in situations where no fundal view is possible. Additionally, it is of particular importance in the setting of ocular oncology for characterising lesion dimensions. In this chapter we provide an overview of the different techniques used and their indications. However, the best method for learning ophthalmic ultrasound is to practise this non-invasive technique on patients.

INDICATIONS

In any situation where there is no clear fundal view, ultrasound provides a useful assessment of the intraocular anatomy. It is worth having a low threshold for undertaking an ultrasound scan. For example, in cases of angle closure or rubeotic glaucoma, where corneal oedema can obscure a proper fundal assessment, ultrasound can be useful for ruling out masses in the vitreous/posterior segment that may be contributing to the development of a secondary angle closure.

Ultrasound is essential in cases where there is no fundal view and surgical intervention, most commonly cataract surgery, is planned. For example, a white cataract may be secondary to a longstanding detached retina or intraocular tumour.

TECHNICAL ASPECTS

Ultrasound uses piezoelectricity to generate sound waves in the probe head. This sound wave is reflected back when travelling through different density tissues. The echo is transduced and amplified to produce peaks corresponding to differing reflective characteristics of ocular tissue.

A (amplitude) scans are a measure of amplitude of returned echo signal over time. The peaks of reflected echoes occur at changes in tissue density. It is therefore a one-dimensional map of the eye. There should be five clear peaks which are outlined in Figure 30.1. The A scan is particularly useful when overlaid on a B (brightness) scan as it can tell you about the internal structure of masses on B scan, to help diagnose a lesion.

The peaks of the A waves in different meridians can be plotted to create the B scan, which is recognisable as a black and white image of the globe itself.

The gain of the B scan can be adjusted to create brighter or darker images. Higher gain is useful for looking at vitreous, but

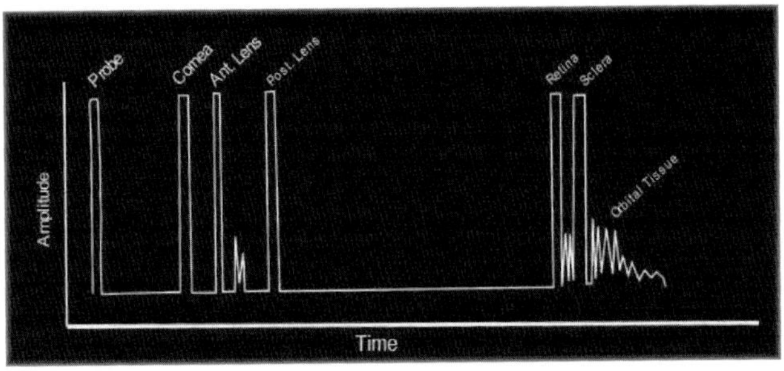

Fig. 30.1 The typical peaks of an A scan, associated with changes in tissue density as a sound wave travels through the eye and is reflected to the probe.

can lose some of the finer retinal detail. Lower gain is used to look for more subtle pathology.

PRACTICAL CONSIDERATIONS

Ultrasound is safe to perform. However, it is best avoided in situations where there is a risk of inducing infection, e.g. early post-operative patients. Additionally, in cases where an open globe is suspected, it is best to avoid ultrasound. It is however possible to perform ultrasound without putting any pressure on the globe. This can be achieved by asking the patient to close their eyes and applying copious amounts of gel over the eyelid, then submerging the probe in this mound of gel without putting pressure on the globe. However, this then needs to be cleared away with no pressure on the eye. Usually, CT scans of the orbits are used to define ocular injury in the setting of a suspected penetrating trauma rather than ultrasound.

For performing ultrasound in routine settings, it can be done either in an anaesthetised eye with direct scleral contact or through a closed eyelid with ultrasound gel applied to the lid. Ultrasound gel can sting and is often not clean enough to directly instill into the eye if a scleral technique is used. A carbomer gel is a better medium. Scleral contact ultrasound is considered to give better image definition as the interference of the lid and lens is not present.

ORIENTATING THE B SCAN

Understanding this is crucial for accurate documentation of findings. Most ultrasound machines use a pencil-like probe with a marker. This marker is where the superior aspect of the image is, so is usually orientated upwards. Some ultrasound machines use the general ultrasound probes which are rectangular in shape and have a similar marking on one side. Their shape does make them less optimal for ophthalmic use.

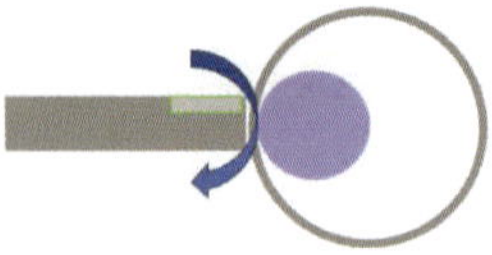

Fig. 30.2A Axial 12.

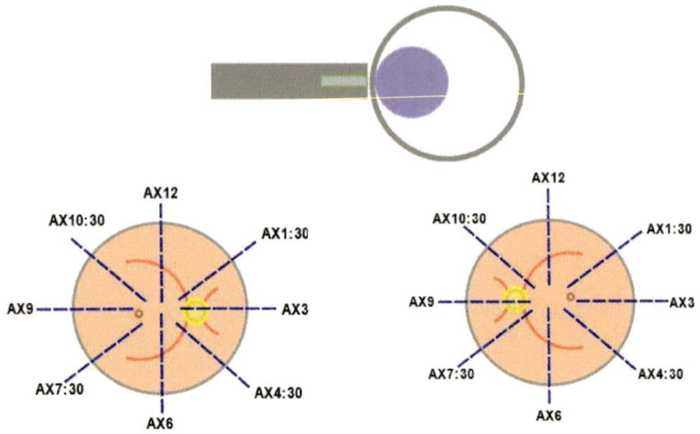

Fig. 30.2B Axial scan planes.

Sections: Axial

The probe sits on top of the cornea with the patient looking straight ahead. As you rotate the probe clockwise, sections of the posterior pole will be taken.

Figure 30.2A shows the probe orientation for the axial 12 scan (marker upwards at 12 o'clock) when rotated clockwise the below diagram (Figure 30.2B) shows axial 3.

In Figure 30.2B, blue lines show the axis along which the axial length scan will lie. The axial scan provides a limited view that does not extend beyond the retinal equator so these diagrams are purely to demonstrate the position of the slices. As you can see, the slices are named after clock hours with intermediate "half past" clock hours present at oblique slices.

Longitudinal

Figure 30.3 shows probe position for a left eye longitudinal scan. The marker is kept facing towards the examiner (who is

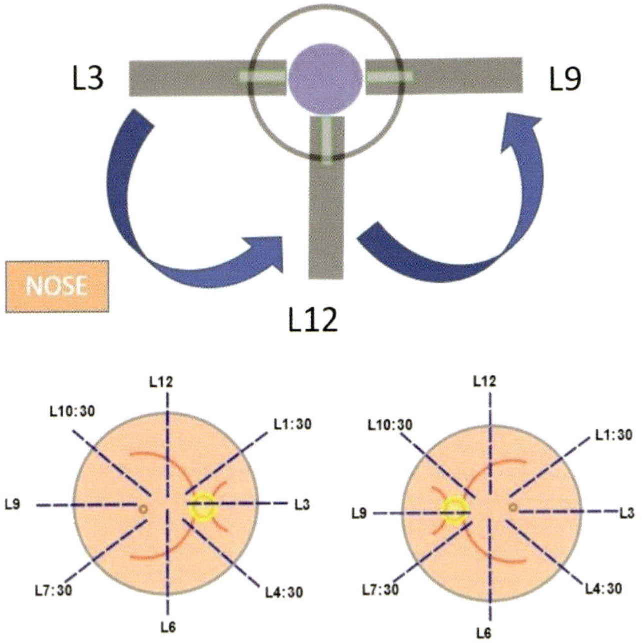

Fig. 30.3 Longitudinal scan planes.

standing in front of the patient) and the probe placed at the limbus. Longitudinal scans of the macula will be obtained when the probe is placed at the nasal limbus. Disc sections are obtained with the probe at the temporal limbus. For the right eye the macula section is L9 but for the left eye it is L3. For the disc section, the converse applies. Longitudinal scans are useful for measuring antero-posterior dimensions of intraocular masses. When measuring lesions, it is important to mention which slice the measurements apply to. Sometimes the measurements are taken to include the sclera or are taken up to the scleral margin. If you can leave the callipers on your ultrasound printout, then this doesn't have to be written but can be useful to explicitly state if callipers cannot be displayed.

Transverse

Transverse scans are best for screening as they cover multiple clock hours of the retina. The patient looks towards the direc-

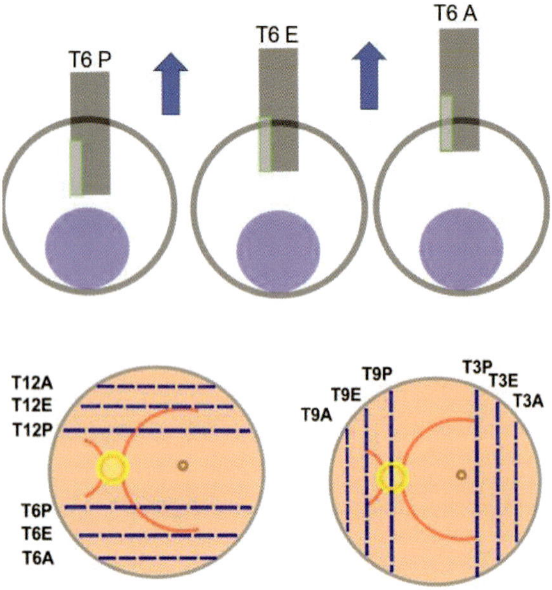

Fig. 30.4 Transverse imaging planes.

tion of the retina you want to scan. In Figure 30.4 the patient is looking down to scan the inferior retina. The marker should be facing nasally when scanning the vertical quadrants. When scanning the horizontal quadrants, the probe marker should be upright. The probe itself is moved from near the limbus back towards the face, following the curve of the sclera. The further back the probe travels, the more anterior the slice. Transverse slices are labelled not just by the clock hour but also by the antero-posterior position: posterior, equatorial, anterior. This allows a subsequent examiner to easily locate pathology you may have found.

Note that T3P for the right eye and T9P for the left eye offer a good section through the optic nerve head.

PERFORMING AN ULTRASOUND B SCAN

Below is a basic screening ultrasound examination which is often done to check that the retina is flat, or that there is no pathology present when no fundal view is present.

Basic ultrasound exam (assuming we are scanning a RIGHT eye):

1. Enter patient details and eye to be scanned onto system, if multiple modes available select B scan.
2. Ensure that the probe is clean.
3. Keep the probe cable out of the way by passing this over your head so it is resting on your shoulders.
4. Apply topical anaesthetic to the sclera if using a scleral contact approach; not needed if you are scanning over lid.
5. Usually, there is a foot pedal to depress, which will start image acquisition; pressing again will freeze the image.
6. Assuming that the patient has their eyes closed and we are scanning over lid, first ask the patient to imagine they are looking straight ahead and take a scan through the primary position with the marker upright (axial 12).
7. Then ask the patient to look to their right and place the probe on the nasal aspect of the eye; the further you move the probe towards the patient's face, the more anterior the ultrasound will scan (T9).
8. The opposite is repeated with the patient looking to their left and scanning the temporal aspect of the same eye (T3).
9. The patient then looks up and the probe is held with the marker facing towards the patient's nose (T12).
10. The patient then looks down and the probe is held with the marker facing nasally again (T6).
11. A macula scan is obtained by placing the probe at the nasal limbus with the marker facing towards you (L9). The eye is looking slightly temporally. You should see the optic nerve at the bottom of the screen and the body of the lateral rectus muscle at the top of the screen. The macula is in between these structures.
12. At all steps you can turn the gain up and down to focus on vitreous or retinal pathology.
13. As well as taking images, pay attention to the way the structures move inside the eye, which is dynamic scanning.

The above is a good retinal screening sequence for any vitreo-retinal abnormalities. It doesn't matter which order you scan around the eye in so long as you can remember the path you take. Note that most of the scans are transverse to cover the retina.

Dynamic Scanning

A retinal detachment and vitreous detachment can sometimes look similar. However, holding the probe on the eye and observing how the detached area moves whilst the patient makes horizontal or vertical saccades can help you decide. A vitreous detachment moves freely, whereas a retinal detachment is less motile. A choroidal detachment (Figure 30.5) has a bulging inward appearance and is non-motile, but can look similar to a retinal detachment due to the thick hyperechogenic layer.

The Importance of A Scan in Diagnosing Intraocular Masses

A scans are particularly useful when faced with an evident mass on B scan. The amount of internal reflectivity (i.e. how much echo is reflected) is a reflection of the irregularity of the internal structure of the tumour so from A scan alone one can infer the type of tumour present.

Figure 30.6 shows high internal reflectivity, the spikes between the retinal and scleral spikes remain high in amplitude.

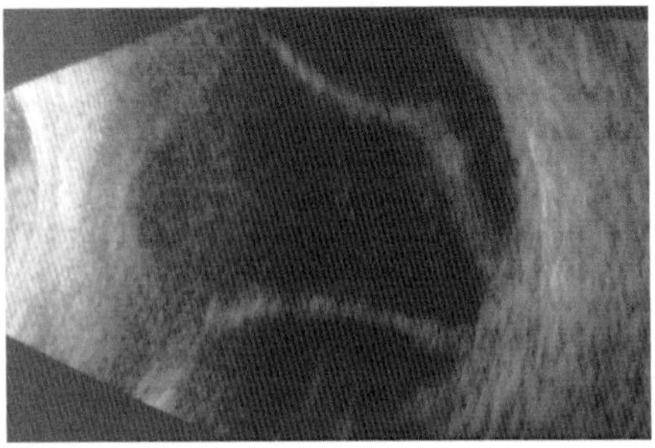

Fig. 30.5 A choroidal detachment caused by an effusion from hypotony. Note the smooth-contoured hyperechogenic line bowing inwards.

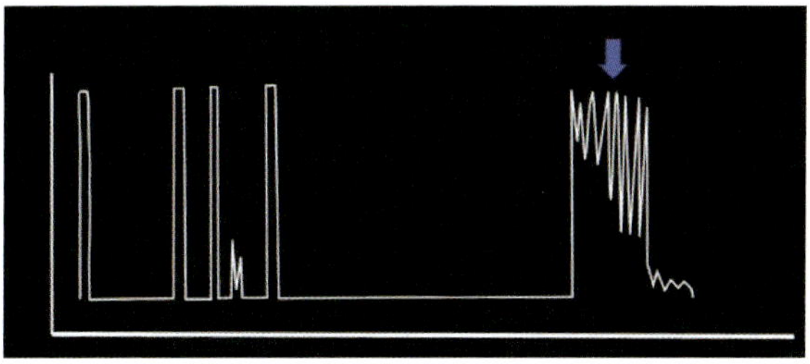

Fig. 30.6 A choroidal lesion with high internal reflectivity.

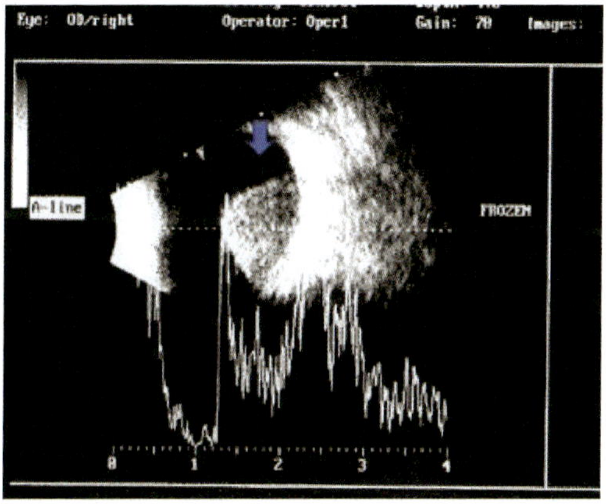

Fig. 30.7 A choroidal melanoma showing low internal reflectivity. Melanomas can also show choroidal excavation and cast a shadow into the orbital structures.

This indicates an irregular internal structure. High internal reflectivity is seen in choroidal haemangiomas most typically. It can also be seen in some metastatic tumours where there is a medium-high internal reflectivity.

Figure 30.7 shows an A scan superimposed on a B scan demonstrating low internal reflectivity (arrow) corresponding with a large dome-shaped lesion on the B scan. This is typical of a choroidal melanoma which has a regular internal structure and so is not as echogenic. Choroidal naevi usually have medium-high internal reflectivity.

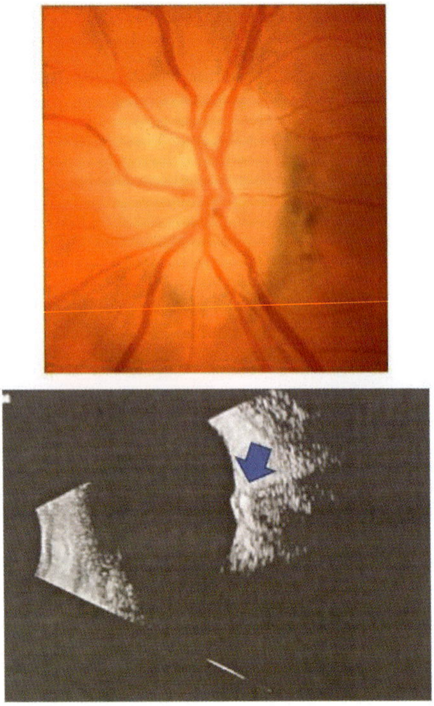

Fig. 30.8 Hyperechogenic drusen in the optic nerve head on ultrasound with corresponding disc photograph.

Optic Nerve Head Ultrasound

Ultrasound of the optic nerve head can be useful for looking for drusen (Figure 30.8) which are best seen with a low gain. They are highly echogenic due to their calcium component.

Ultrasound can also be used to assess disc swelling caused by other causes. When a transverse section through the optic nerve is taken (as shown in Figure 30.9) dark fluid can be seen either side of the optic nerve head if swelling is present. Where fluid surrounds the nerve, it can lead to a "donut" or "crescent" sign depending on how much fluid is present. The nerve diameter with the surrounding fluid can be measured with callipers, which then forms the basis of the 30° test. This distinguishes between solid swelling and fluid within the optic nerve sheath.

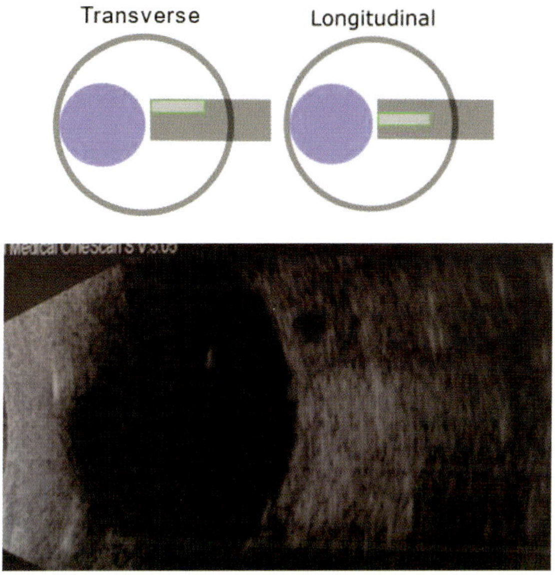

Fig. 30.9 The hypoechogenic nerve head is seen in transverse section, which is captured by placing the probe temporally against the limbus with the marker upright (transverse orientation). This is showing a left eye with gaze directed nasally.

The probe is held temporally, obtaining a transverse image and the patient then looks towards it at about 30°. This puts the optic nerve on tension and redistributes the fluid along the length of the nerve, resulting in a decrease in nerve sheath width. Where this reduction is >15% the test is said to be positive, suggesting a diagnosis of raised intracranial pressure.[1]

Biometry

As detailed in the biometry chapter, biometry is usually conducted via optical means nowadays. Historically, A scan ultrasounds were used to determine axial length. Then keratometry was performed separately on a dedicated keratometer. It is still occasionally necessary to perform biometry in this way, most commonly in cases where the cataract is too dense to permit optic recording of the axial length. Here, an ultrasound probe

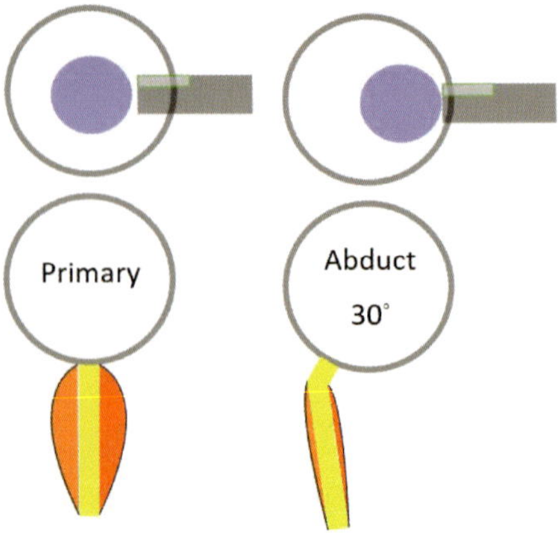

Fig. 30.10 In the 30° test (of a left eye here) the participant abducts their eye by 30° from the primary position whilst the probe is kept on the eye temporally. A decrease in the sheath diameter is seen as fluid is redistributed along the optic nerve from the nerve being placed on tension.

(usually one dedicated purely to biometry recordings) is utilised. Keratometry can be performed using a handheld keratometer (e.g. Nidek HandyRef-K) or taken from the IOLMaster biometry machine.

Great care must be taken when taking ultrasound readings using an A scan probe as indentation of the cornea can falsely shorten the axial length. Additionally, the gates and thresholds must be set correctly to ensure accurate readings.

Gates are markers (also known as cursors) which allow the machine to detect the four key peaks (cornea, anterior lens, posterior lens, retina). These peaks are used to determine axial length. As Figure 30.1 shows, there is noise in between these peaks, so a threshold sensitivity has to be set as well to signify which amplitude is significant. Gates are marked just before the four peaks and the machine will then detect a peak to the right of this that is above threshold. This will then be registered as the peak for the relevant anatomical structure. Although the machine will automatically generate gates, they may need to be adjusted, for example to account for lens thickness. Aphakic patients should have the lens gates removed.

These gates need to be checked for accuracy if manual biometry is being performed as errors may result in incorrect axial length measurement. A corneal gate too far right or a retinal gate too far left well result in overly myopic outcomes. This is due to the machine registering the eye as smaller, recommending a more powerful lens than required, which then results in the focal point being anterior to the retina. Immersion ultrasound (where the probe is submerged in a pool of water sitting on top of the eye) is the gold standard for A scan biometry. However, it is cumbersome and requires specialist training.

ULTRASOUND BIOMICROSCOPY (UBM)

UBM is used for visualising the anterior chamber and is particularly useful for examining the ciliary body as the iris blocks optical imaging techniques of this structure [for example, Figure 30.11 shows a ciliary body cyst that was not visible on optical coherence tomography (OCT)]. Its uses high frequencies of around 50 MHz to provide short-range penetration into the

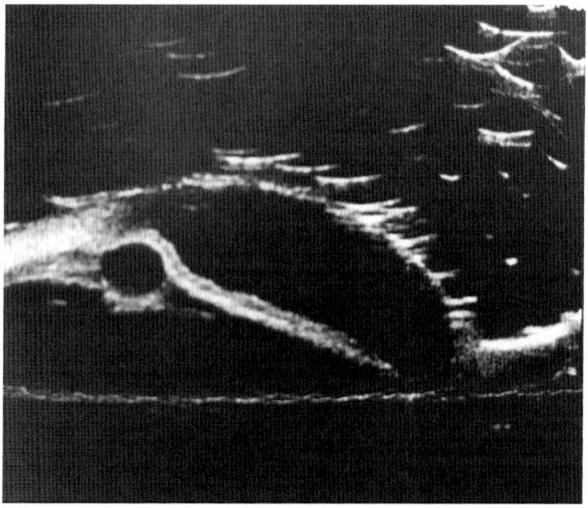

Fig. 30.11 Ciliary body cyst seen causing forward bowing of the iris in a transverse section.

eye, which allows good visualisation of anterior and posterior chamber structures. The probe will visualise the structures closest to it when taking slices. Therefore, transverse scans image the ciliary body and processes well. You can even make out zonular detail. Axial scans give a good view of the lens and anterior chamber generally and the angle is best visualised with longitudinal slices.

UBM differs from conventional ultrasound in that it contains a probe head which requires submersion in water to achieve adequate scans. You cannot use gel with UBM; instead a probe cover is usually provided which is filled with water and fixed around the probe to provide a watertight seal. This is then directly applied onto an anaesthetised eye.

CONCLUSIONS

Ultrasound is an essential skill that should be used in almost every case of no fundal view being present but especially pre-cataract surgery and in dense vitreous haemorrhages. A screening technique is important to know and be adept at, to quickly rule out pathology in such settings. Learning the terminology for documenting slice orientation is particularly important when lesions are measured for continuing surveillance, e.g. intraocular tumours, choroidal naevi.

Reference

1. Kyung SR, Wall P, Hayden B, Rychwalski P. (2013) The accuracy of the 30 Degree Test in Detecting Increased Intracranial Pressure When Compared to CSF Opening Pressure on Lumbar Puncture. *Invest Ophthalmol Vis Sci* **54**(15): 2314.

31

CORNEAL TOMOGRAPHY

Thomas Sherman

INTRODUCTION

We can inspect the cornea with the slit lamp to determine if there are any visible structural abnormalities and we can also refract the patient to deduce what prescription their glasses should be. However, these investigations do not provide a detailed assessment of shape of the cornea, which is key to understanding its refractive properties.

A tomograph is a representation of a three-dimensional solid structure that details the object's internal structure. This contrasts with a topograph, which is a representation of the surface features of an object. Nowadays, the corneal tomograph (most commonly generated by the Pentacam® device) is more common than topographs. However, you may occasionally encounter historic topographs (e.g. Orbscan®). We will not discuss analysis of topographs due to their infrequent use. However, the most important point is that you cannot directly compare a topography printout with a tomography printout.

How does corneal tomography work?

The crucial component of the Pentacam® is its rotating Scheimpflug camera, with a second camera detecting residual eye movements. The Pentacam® produces a slit illumination of the cornea which needs to be captured by a camera that can ensure that every point of the image, at all distances from the lens, is perfectly in focus. This is achieved with the Scheimpflug method, explained in Figure 31.1. The Pentacam® takes 50–100 images in 2 seconds, depending on the model used, with up to 138,000 analysable points.[1] There is no contact with the eye and no need for the patient to have any anaesthetic drops put in. Sometimes, if a patient's ocular surface is particularly dry,

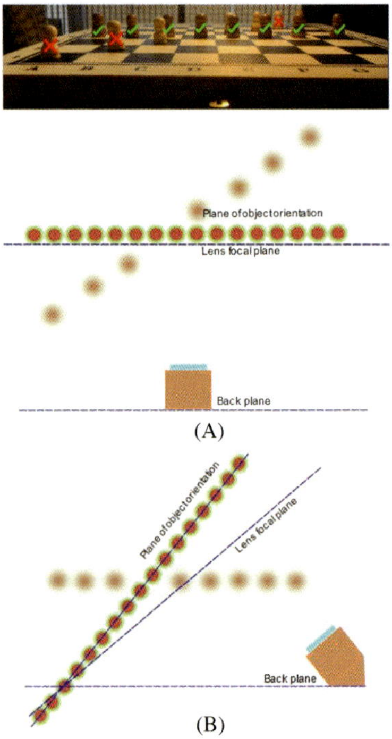

Fig. 31.1 (A) The plane of focus is parallel to the lens plane in a camera. So the chess board with the lens facing straight on will have all the dark figures in focus. However, the white figures not parallel to the lens are out of focus. The blue lines show the lens plane and back plane (where the camera sensor is located) orientation. The diagram looks at the camera-object setup from a bird's eye view. (B) When the lens plane is tilted but not parallel to the object plane, then the back plane, object plane and lens plane will intersect. This creates an image with near and distant areas in focus. This is needed to image the close and distant aspects of the cornea, as if you were imaging the side of a hill.

this may reduce the quality of the scan, so instilling a few drops of saline can help improve image quality. Viscous artificial tears may disrupt some of the readings obtained, so are best avoided.

Why is corneal tomography necessary?

Quantifying the three-dimensional structure of the cornea is important for three principal reasons:

1. Diagnosing ectatic disease (disorder of corneal thickness and shape).
2. Monitoring ectatic disease for progression.
3. Planning corneal refractive interventions.

The intention of this chapter is to provide a basic introduction in interpreting tomography. However, the focus of interpreting a tomograph varies depending on what question you need to answer. We will focus on Pentacam® interpretation as this is the most commonly used device. Other brands are also available, as Figure 31.2 shows.

For most of these purposes we are making sense of astigmatism. It is worth being familiar with the basic principles of this.

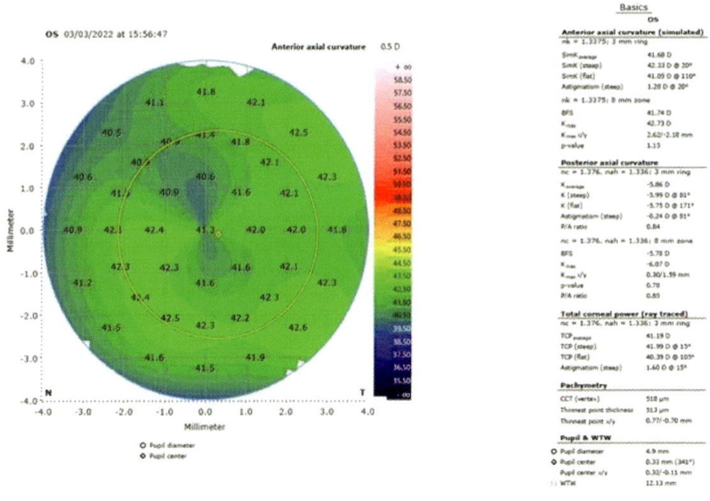

Fig. 31.2 Tomography readout from the Heidelberg Anterion® device, which as you will see later incorporates many similar indices to Pentacam® measurements.

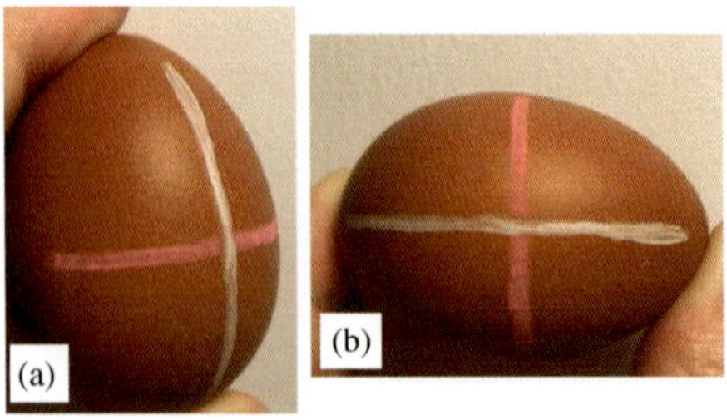

Fig. 31.3 Egg curvature.

The cornea is not a perfect dome shape. It is an ellipse, longer in its horizontal diameter than vertical. Due to this, it has a steep curve and a less steep curve in two different directions. Figure 31.3 outlines this using an egg to show the steep and shallow curves it has.

The pink line on the egg shows its steep curve and the white line shows its shallow curve. I have photographed the egg from the side to exaggerate the curvature. You can see that the steep curve has two orientations, in B it is vertical in A it is horizontal. The orientation is termed the meridian when referring to corneal anatomy. The cornea, like the egg, has a steep and flat meridian. To correct refractive error from a steep meridian, a cylinder lens is used. This must be placed at a particular orientation, termed its axis. Meridian is the correct term to use when referring to corneal shape, but often people use the term axis.[2] Usually, the steep and flat meridians are 90° from each other, which is termed regular astigmatism. Regular astigmatism is either with the rule (steep axis vertical), against the rule (steep axis horizontal) or oblique (steep axis is diagonal). Egg B shows with the rule astigmatism. It needs a corrective positive cylindrical lens placed at a 90° axis. Egg A shows against the rule astigmatism. It needs a corrective positive cylindrical lens placed at a 180° axis. Where the steep meridian is not 90° to the flat meridian, this is termed irregular astigmatism. Irregular astigmatism occurs in corneal ectasia, following corneal grafts or trauma.

How do I use the information gathered?

Large amounts of data are gathered when the Pentacam® scan has finished, and there are multiple maps which display this data. Maps are reports produced by the Pentacam® software that display key indices of relevance to the clinical questions. In most cases the question we are answering is "Is there ectasia?" or "Is there progression of ectasia?" and the maps most commonly used for these purposes are the four map refractive readout and the Belin Ambrosio display. We will focus on interpreting these two maps.

What should I check first on these maps?

Like any report, check if the patient information is correct and that you are looking at the report from the correct date. Check the quality specifications; black dots around the edge of the map signify areas of poor quality and a yellow shading to the QS box (Figure 31.4) signifies significant quality issues with the scan. There are usually some black dots in the periphery,

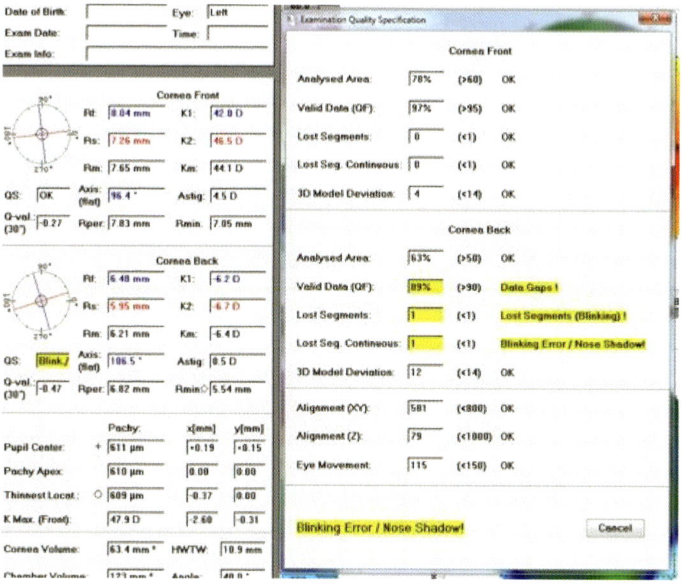

Fig. 31.4 This display is obtained by clicking on the yellow box and tells you the exact fields that were disrupted, in this case by blinking. You can gauge the magnitude of the deviation from optimal conditions, which in this case was not particularly high and only applied to readings of the back surface of the cornea.

which do not negate the scan. The QS box will guide you more about whether the scan is acceptable or not. If yellow, it may be worth repeating the scan. Bear in mind that fluorescein causes significant back scattering and can impede quality.

There are different settings that can be altered by more advanced Pentacam users. It is worth checking what typical settings your clinic uses. The colour scale used in our figures is Belin intuitive (dark red to purple). For ectasia purposes you usually select an 8 mm best fit sphere (BFS) setting (sometimes optometrists may change this to best fit toric ellipsoid when dealing with contact lens prescriptions), which we will discuss the meaning of later.

Note that QS is a measure of quality, but Q-Val is a measure of the overall sphericity of the cornea.

INTERPRETING A FOUR MAPS REFRACTIVE PRINTOUT

The four maps (Figure 31.5) are:

- Front curvature
- Front elevation
- Back elevation
- Corneal thickness

As you can see, there is much information provided here. It is helpful to breakdown what each of these segments means. However, you are highly unlikely to use all these values, so this is just for reference purposes. Highlighted in red in each image are the particularly useful/important parameters.

Cornea Front and Back Keratometry Values

There are two separate boxes for front (Figure 31.6) and back (Figure 31.7) corneal surfaces, as the curvature of these two may be different from one another.

The map on the left shows the orientation of the flat meridian (flat meridian is always K1). In this case 65°. The red line

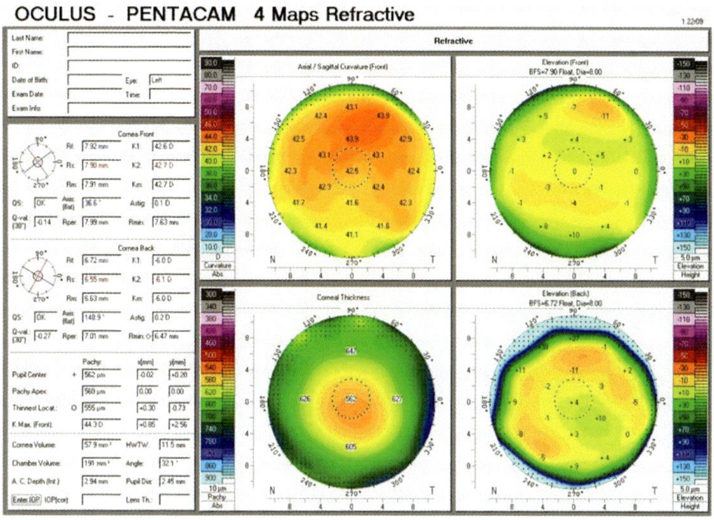

Fig. 31.5 A typical four maps refractive printout with no ectasia.

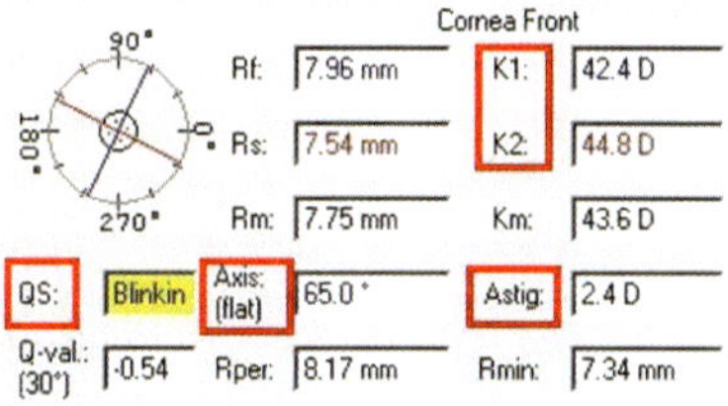

Fig. 31.6 Front keratometry values.

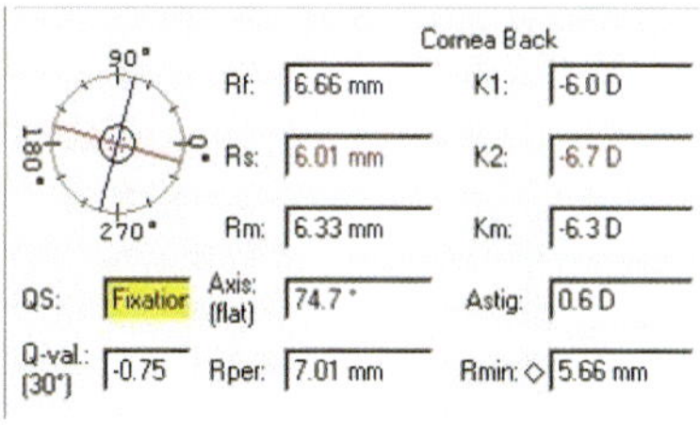

Fig. 31.7 Back keratometry values.

shows the steep meridian (K2) which is 90° from K1. Rf and Rs (flat and steep) represent the radii of curvature. We don't tend to use these but rather the K values given in dioptres. A normal K value should be below 47.2 dioptres (D) and in keratoconus is usually >48.7 D. Rper is the average radius of curvature between the 6 mm and 9 mm zone centre and Rmin, the smallest radius of curvature. Again these are not used as frequently as K values. Astig refers to the central corneal astigmatism measured in dioptres and is the difference between K1 and K2. Q-Val has been previously mentioned as a measure of asphericity. It should be between −1 and 0 with less than −1 indicating possible ectasia.

Note that these measurements are repeated for the back corneal surface, which has negative K values.

Pachymetric Indices With Co-Ordinates

Pachymetry measures corneal thickness. The normal range from central corneal thickness is 540–560 µm. The pachymetry of the corneal apex is the reference point by which the other pachymetric indices are orientated. The X (horizontal) and Y (vertical) values signify the mm by which the points vary from this reference, for both the thinnest location and the pachymetry over the pupil centre. The difference between the geometric central point and the thinnest point of the cornea is higher in keratoconus cases.

The Kmax of the corneal front curvature is widely used for judging keratoconus progression and response to corneal cross-linking. It represents the steepest area of anterior curvature and a Kmax increase of 1D or more from baseline is defined as

		Pachy:	x[mm]	y[mm]
Pupil Center:	+	579 µm	-0.41	-0.06
Pachy Apex:	·	588 µm	0.00	0.00
Thinnest Locat.:	O	568 µm	-1.68	-0.25
K Max. (Front):		46.0 D	+2.18	-0.62

Fig. 31.8 Pachymetric indices with co-ordinates.

progression of keratoconus. However, Kmax does have limitations in that it doesn't reflect the degree of ectasia, ignores any contribution of the posterior cornea to progression and progression can occur with no changes in Kmax.[3]

Other Values

The bottom panel of the four maps refractive printout contains data about the corneal volume and anterior chamber characteristics. HWTW is horizontal white to white. These do not tend to be utilised widely in the cornea clinic but can be useful in a glaucoma context.

Maps

Anterior corneal curvature is shown in Figure 31.9, where cool colours show flatter curvature and hotter colours show steeper curvature. Note the black dots in the periphery indicating suboptimal scan quality in these areas.

The N and T orientate the cornea to nasal and temporal. The axis lines with a central point of 0 out to 8 demark the concentric rings in mm outwards from the central point. Note that actually a 9 mm total diameter is scanned. For more peripheral ectasias, sometimes it is necessary to examine out at

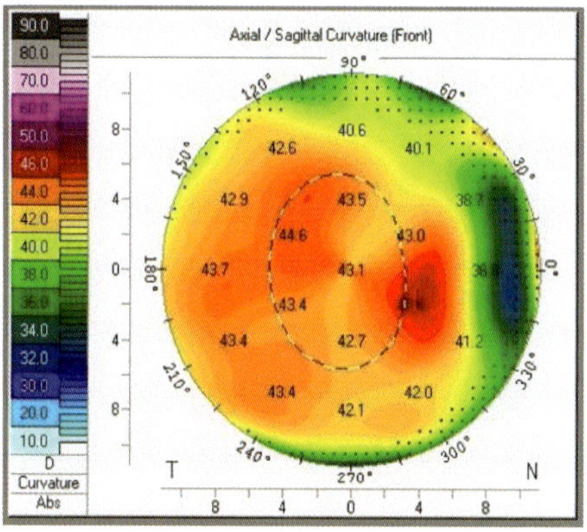

Fig. 31.9 Front curvature map.

12 mm, e.g. pellucid marginal degeneration. The numeric values are the K values in dioptres at these points.

Regular astigmatism shows up on this map as a "bow tie" appearance. If this bow tie is vertical, there is with the rule astigmatism and horizontal means against the rule. Where there is a symmetric bow tie, it represents regular astigmatism.

You can see in Figure 31.9 that there is a bow tie appearance horizontally but it has some degree of asymmetry. This indicates irregular astigmatism and possibly an ectasia, though this was not the case in this person's scan.

The anterior curvature map is limited in diagnosing keratoconus as it is just providing us with absolute K values (dotted around the map), rather than telling us how much the cornea departs from an expected spherical shape, which is what the two elevation maps tell us.

Elevation Maps (Front and Back)

The elevation maps for the front and back curvature of the cornea are based on the same important principle of a BFS. This provides a more sensitive way of detecting corneal ectasia than relying on absolute K values.

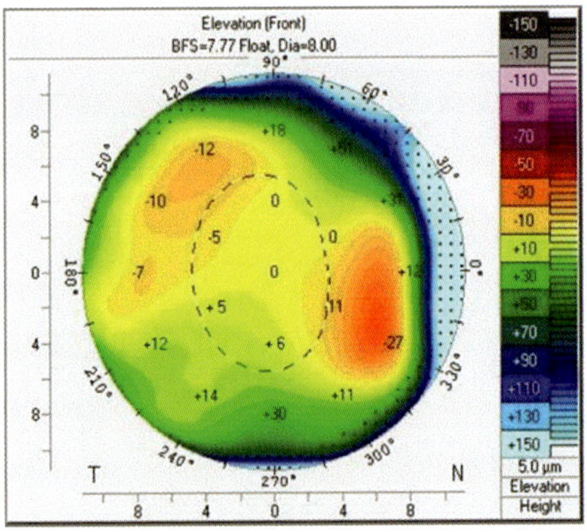

Fig. 31.10 Front elevation map.

What is BFS?

The BFS is a geometric concept. It is a sphere that when superimposed on the measured cornea produces the least amount of residuals (i.e. deviations from this geometrically optimal sphere). There will always be some points above and below the sphere. The heat map shows how much individual points on the cornea depart from the BFS, with cooler colours above the BFS and warmer colours below the BFS.

In Figure 31.11 the blue-shaded semicircle is the BFS. The red line above is the flat axis. Its curve is broader and less steep than the BFS. The dark blue line is the steep axis, which is mostly below the BFS. Imagine that the semicircle diagram is looking at the BFS side on.

In the elevation map, cool colours signify that the cornea is above the BFS (just as cool colours on the curvature map indicate less curvature) but warmer colours indicate that the curvature is below the BFS (more curved). The diagram below the BFS in Figure 31.11 shows how the dark purple colour is seen along the dark blue line, indicating the point at maximal depression below the BFS. The converse colour pattern applies

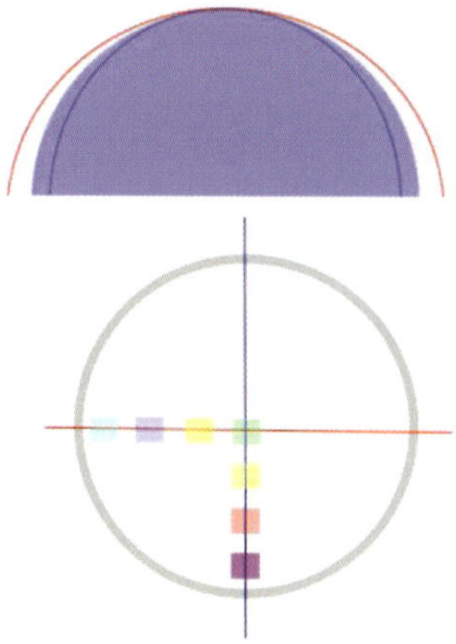

Fig. 31.11 The concept of BFS and colour examples at different points.

for the red line above the BFS. Centrally, both lines do not depart much from the BFS, so become yellow/green.

The BFS is applied as a "float" which simply means that there are not positioning restraints on where the BFS can be fitted. The BFS is applied to an 8 mm area, although as you saw previously, a wider area is measured.

Hotspots indicate areas of greater curvature in a particular location which may indicate an ectasia is present (Figure 31.12). In a normal cornea, the majority of the elevation map is green with some peripheral red or blue areas. In keratoconus, the back surface is affected early, so early-stage keratoconus may be diagnosed on the basis of an abnormal back elevation map, whilst the rest of the cornea appears more normally curved.

Pachymetry Map

Eyes with keratoconus have a thinner cornea and at the apex of the cone will have an area of maximal thinning. Thinner areas

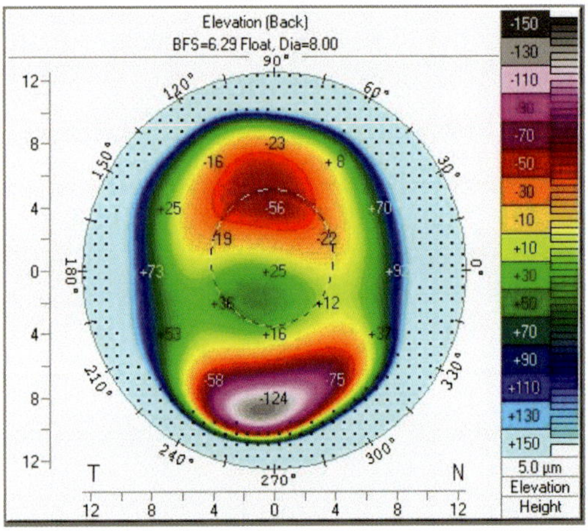

Fig. 31.12 This back elevation map is taken from a patient with keratoconus. Inferiorly, you can see a black/purple area which is severely depressed below the BFS, i.e. very curved. There is then a sharp change back to being elevated above the BFS peripherally. Note that a 12 mm area has been measured but the BFS is applied to an 8 mm diameter area.

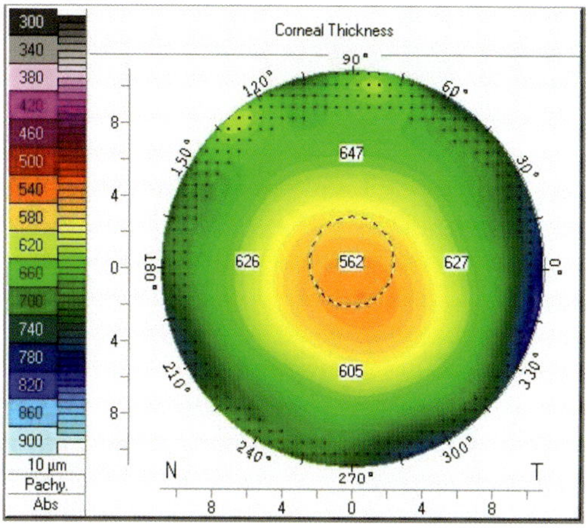

Fig. 31.13 Pachymetry map in a normal eye.

are displayed as warmer colours on the pachymetry map. Figure 31.13 shows a normal cornea where the thinnest point is present centrally.

Summary Four Map Refractive

- Check patient information and date of scan correct
- Check K1, K2, axis and astigmatism
- Look at anterior curvature map for evidence of irregularity (asymmetric bow tie)
- Look for any hotspots on the elevation maps (back and front)

INTERPRETING A BELIN AMBROSIO ENHANCED ECTASIA DISPLAY (BAD)

The BAD is geared specifically at keratoconus diagnosis and monitoring. It consists of:

- Elevation front maps
- Elevation back maps

- Keratometry, pachymetry and progression indices
- Mean corneal thickness graphs
- Corneal thickness display

Like the four maps refractive layout, there are many parameters displayed. Abnormal values will display red or yellow. I focus more on what these various parameters mean rather than providing normal ranges, which can be found in the Pentacam® manual and literature put out by Oculus, the company that manufactures the device.

Elevation Front Maps

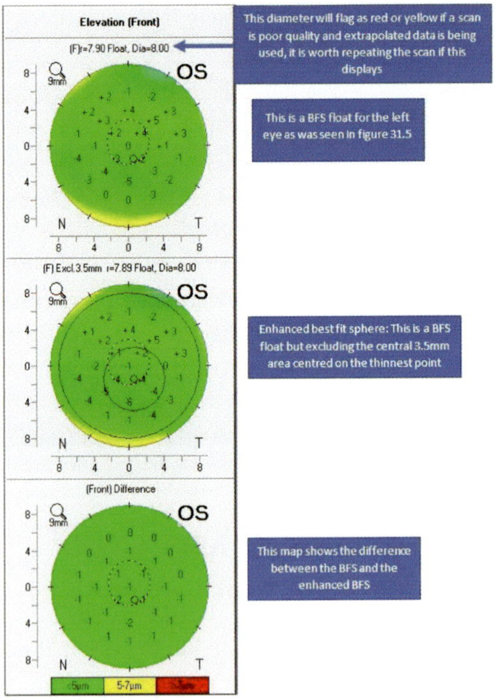

Fig. 31.14 Front elevation maps for BAD in a cornea with no ectasia.

Why exclude an area centred on thinnest point?

When a BFS is applied to a cornea with keratoconus, the abnormal cone will contribute data points that will then be used to fit the sphere. The problem here is that it will camouflage the abnormal cone area by fitting a sphere skewed by the abnormally steep readings. By excluding the thinnest point and an area 4 mm around it, the cone is removed from calculating the BFS and so will be displayed much more prominently as a hot spot. This map offers improved sensitivity on the standard BFS float. The difference map then exaggerates the difference between the two maps to make the cone more noticeable, a difference of more than 12 μm for the front elevation and 20 μm for back elevation are abnormal.[4]

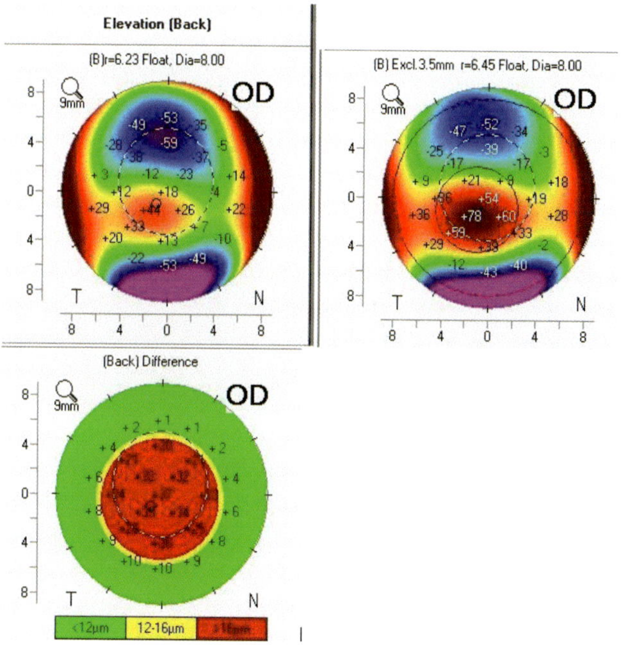

Fig. 31.15 Back elevation maps for an eye with keratoconus. In the elevation map there is an inferior hot spot that then becomes much more pronounced in the exclusion map, with the hotspot then being even more obvious in the difference map.

Elevation Back Maps

These are of particular interest as keratoconus usually starts by affecting the back curvature of the cornea, so early diagnosis can be achieved by paying particular attention to this map. The layout is the same as the front curvature maps.

Progression Indices and Thickness Display

Most of these indices are familiar from the four maps refractive. However, there are some additions.

Pachymetry at the thinnest point is measured in the direction from the apex (IT indicates that it is displaced in an inferotemporal direction). Studies have shown this value to be higher in keratoconic corneas compared to unaffected eyes.

The thickness map has several rings centred around the thinnest point. The average of thickness values around these rings is then recorded. The coloured lines detail the directions of change in thickness across the cornea. The blue line shows where the change in thickness is most rapid and the green line shows where the change is slowest. These correspond to the progression index min. (green) and max. (blue).

Front elevation at thinnest location and back elevation and thinnest location measure departure from the BFS at these

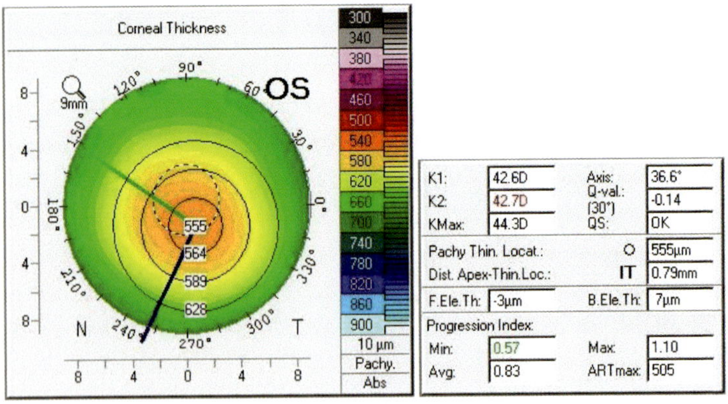

Fig. 31.16 Progression indices and thickness display in an eye with no ectasia.

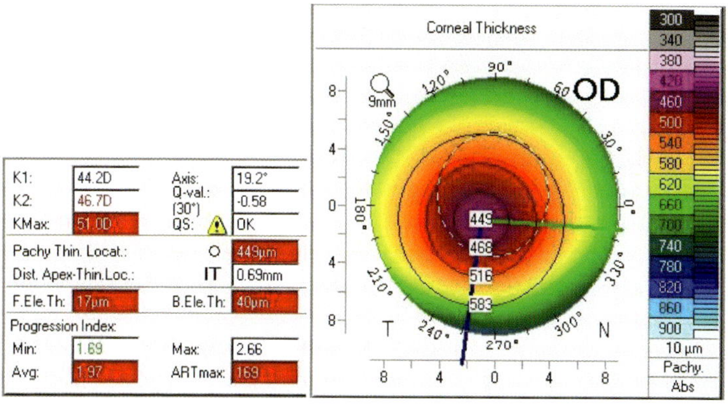

Fig. 31.17 Pachymetric map in a keratoconic eye showing abnormal Kmax, an abnormally thin central cornea and rapid thickness progression inferotemporally. The progression indices show abnormal average progression in thickness across the cornea and abnormal ARTmax.

locations. The ARTmax is the Ambrosio relational thickness, which is the thinnest point divided by the progression index. Where this is low a diagnosis of keratoconus is suggested (Figure 31.17).

Pachymetric Evaluation Graphs

These are graphical representations of the map outlined in the previous section. The thickness data from 22 rings in 0.4 mm steps around the thinnest point are averaged. These are then plotted on a line graph. The X axis corresponds to the ring from which the pachymetric data are obtained and the Y axis is the thickness in micrometres. There are two graphs, corneal thickness spatial profile (CTSP) and percentage thickness increase (PTI) (Figure 31.18).

- CTSP: A normal cornea should become gradually thicker as one progresses further outwards through the concentric rings. Where an ectasia is present, there are abrupt changes that violate this gradual progression. The cornea suddenly becomes thicker moving peripherally from a pathologically thin section to unaffected, normal section of cornea.

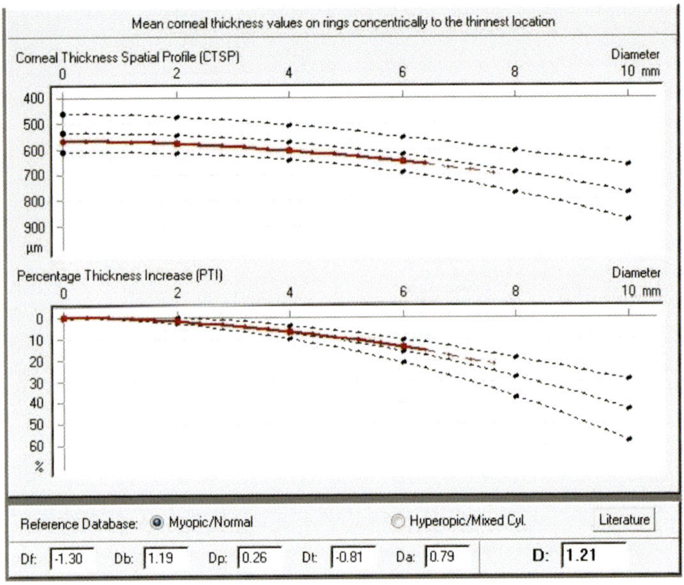

Fig. 31.18 CTSP and PTI graph in an eye with no ectasia. Note the red line stays within the normal confidence intervals.

- PTI: This is effectively the same principle as CTSP but represents the percentage increase in average thickness as you move outward from ring to ring. It can make the deviation easier to gauge than just looking at CTSP.

The mean and two standard deviations are displayed as dashed lines. Where the red line, which is the measured values, veers outside of these standard deviations an ectasia is likely to be present. There are numerous values at the bottom which correspond to:

- Df — Deviation front elevation difference map
- Db — Deviation back elevation difference map
- Dp — Deviation of average pachymetric progression
- Dt — Deviation of minimum thickness
- Da — Deviation of ARTmax (Ambrosio relational thickness)
- D — Total deviation value

Where there is a significant departure from normality (the reference database is held on the machine), the box is flagged. Red boxes indicate that the value is >2.65 SD from mean and yellow are >1.65 SD from the mean. The total deviation value (D) represents a good screening tool as to whether an ectasia may be present.

BAD Summary

- Look for hot spots on the enhanced BFS maps (particularly back surface for early disease) and difference map.
- Look at the D value; if red or yellow then an ectasia may be present.
- Look at the CTSP and PTI; does the red line cross outside of the confidence intervals (Figure 31.19)?

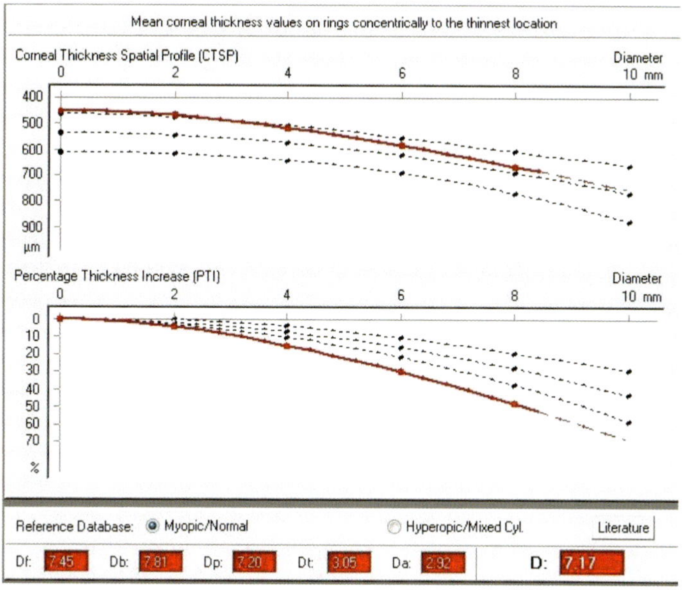

Fig. 31.19 CTSP and PTI in a keratoconic eye. Note the red line is markedly outside the PTI confidence intervals and crosses through the CTSP confidence intervals. The deviation indices are all highly abnormal.

CONCLUSION

Interpretation of corneal tomography is really dependent on what question you are hoping to answer with the data. There are many other maps and applications of the Pentacam® and your corneal specialist may have particular maps or displays they preferentially use. The Pentacam® manual is freely available online and provides an excellent source of further information.

References

1. McAlinden C, Khadka J, Pesudovs K. (2011) A comprehensive evaluation of the precision (repeatability and reproducibility) of the Oculus Pentacam HR. *Invest Ophthalmol Vis Sci* **52**(10): 7731–7737.
2. Rosen E. (2011) Axis or meridian? *J Cataract Refract Surg* **37**(10): 1743.
3. Duncan JK, Belin MW, Borgstrom M. (2016) Assessing progression of keratoconus: novel tomographic determinants. *Eye Vis* **3**(1): 6.
4. Belin MW, Khachikian SS, Salomão M, Ambrósio R Jr. (2011) Keratoconus/ectasia detection with the Oculus Pentacam: Belin/Ambrósio enhanced ectasia display. *Highl Ophthalmol* **35**(6): 5–12.

32

ELECTRODIAGNOSTIC TESTING

Thomas Sherman

Electrodiagnostic testing (EDT) has a reputation of complexity. Indeed it does represent a detailed evaluation of the visual system which has some fascinating physiology that underpins the production of EDT results. The aim of this chapter is to introduce when EDTs tend to be performed, what the different forms of EDTs are, their physiological basis, some common abnormal results and some considerations in their interpretation.

What are Electrodiagnostic Tests?

There are three different tests that are considered under the EDT umbrella:

- Electroretinograms (ERGs)
- Electro-oculograms (EOGs)
- Visual evoked potentials (VEPs)

ERGs are then subdivided into different subtypes which are detailed below.

ELECTRORETINOGRAMS

These are used to examine retinal function, whereas optical coherence tomography (OCT) scans and other imaging of the retina provide details about anatomical integrity from which we deduce the likelihood of functional disruption of the relevant structures. Scans do not in themselves measure how well the structures actually work. That is the missing detail which the ERG informs us of. Accordingly, ERGs may be of particular use where OCT provides limited information about dysfunction of the retina, yet the history (e.g. nyctalopia) or examination findings (e.g. poor acuity, generalised fields construction) suggest that there is organic pathology present. They also represent a useful investigation in assessing people who may be carriers of genetic mutations affecting retinal function, as well as acting as a means of monitoring progression of retinal dysfunction.

There are three types of ERG:

- Full field
- Multifocal
- Pattern

Full field is more widely available than pattern and multifocal ERGs.

Full Field ERGs (ffERGs)

ffERGs measure retinal response to a flash of light. However, this flash of light needs to be carefully standardised, so ffERG uses a Ganzfeld stimulus (Figure 32.1) and requires dilation to ensure that entire retina is illuminated. Ganzfeld means whole field in German and is a specially designed piece of equipment that ensures even illumination across the whole visual field. ffERGs are recorded in light- and dark-adapted states to delineate different photoreceptor responses.

Electrodes are placed with one on the skin and another in direct contact with the eye. Usually, this is a contact lens with a gold electrode, compared to a lid skin electrode. However,

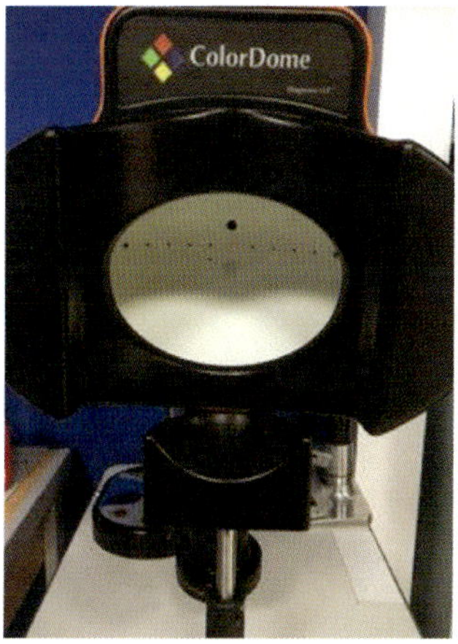

Fig. 32.1 Ganzfeld stimulus. The chinrest and shape of the device means that the entire visual field is evenly illuminated when the patient's face is aligned with the opening.

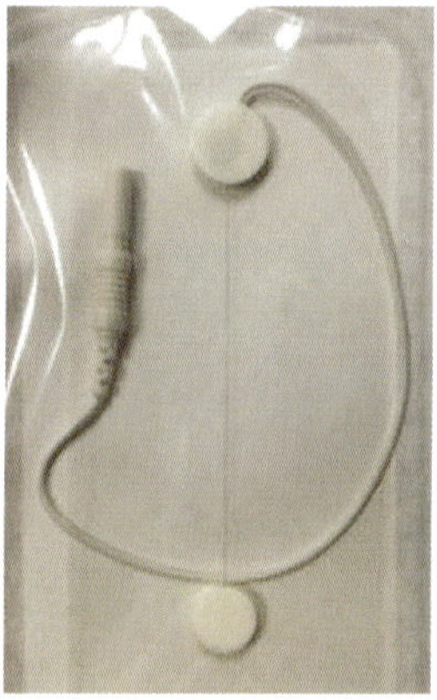

Fig. 32.2 DTL electrode.

eyelid skin electrodes may be used both for reference and for taking measurements, particularly in children. A small thin wire known as a DTL electrode (Figure 32.2) can also be used.

When taking a ffERG, a standard protocol is used called the ISCEV protocol, which can be accessed online. It is summarised below.

ffERG Summary (Figure 32.3)

Dark-Adapted

- DA0.01:
  - o 20 minutes in dark, then a dim flash appears
  - o b- wave only (a- wave may be minimally detectable)
  - o Measures the rod system's general function (abnormality can mean photoreceptor or post-photoreceptor cells are damaged)
- DA3:
  - o Brighter flash (3 cd/m^2 hence DA3)
  - o Mixed rod and cone responses (rod mainly)
  - o Has an a- and b- wave
- DA10:
  - o Brightest flash (10 cd/m^2)
  - o Mixed rod and cone responses (rod mainly)
  - o Has an a- and b- wave
  - o Defines a- wave and rod contribution better than DA3, photoreceptor contribution more well defined

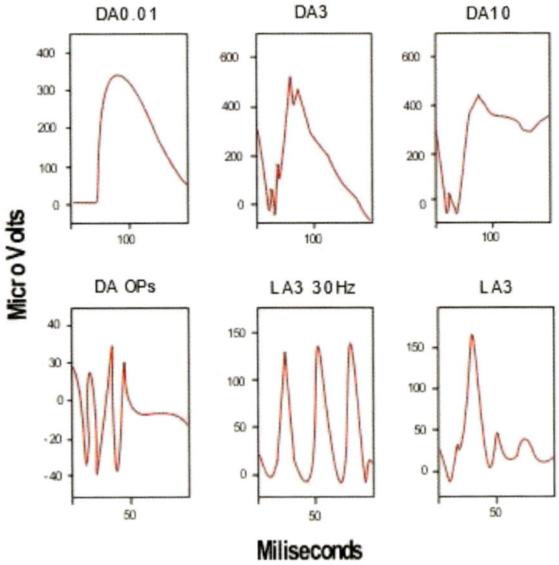

Fig. 32.3 A normal ffERG reported according to the ISCEV protocol.

- DA OP:
  - A more detailed view of the ascending b- wave in bright flash ERGs
  - Generated by amacrine cells
  - Limited clinical utility in isolation but can have relevance in diagnosing certain conditions where other ERGs are abnormal

Light-Adapted

- LA3 30 Hz:
  - 10 minutes of light stimulation in Ganzfeld, then bright (3 cd/m^2) light flickers at 30 Hz
  - Cone responses only (mainly inner cone system)
- LA3:
  - Single bright flash in light-adapted state
  - Has an a- and b- wave
  - Cone responses only
  - Larger amplitude than flicker (assuming no cone disease)

Each of these six bullet points represents six ffERGs. As mentioned, different ERGs measure different photoreceptor systems. The a- and b- waves (Figure 32.4) are important in interpreting ERGs as they derive from different cells:

- a- waves — photoreceptors (rod or cone)
  - This is the first, negative deflection
- b- waves — bipolar cells (pathology suggests inner retinal dysfunction)
  - Positive deflection after the a- wave

The amplitude of the waves is most important, followed by the delay. Pathological states will reduce amplitude and increase delay. There are also c- and d- waves. c- waves arise from the retinal pigment epithelium (RPE) and d- waves arise from OFF bipolar cells. These are not of clinical importance. An important point about light-adapted ERGs is that although they reflect general cone system function, the majority of cones are

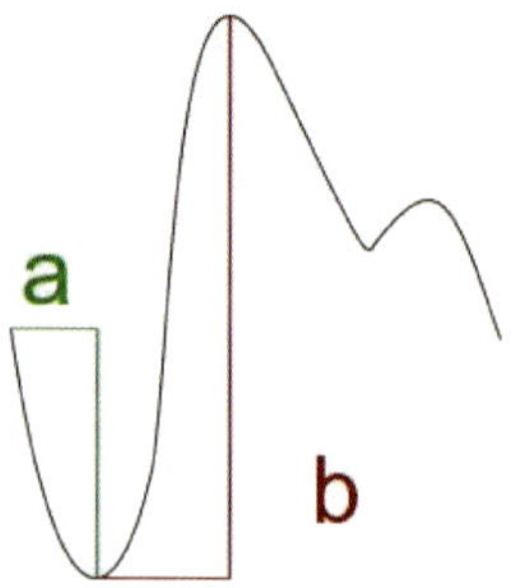

Fig. 32.4 The a- wave delay is measured from onset of flash to the trough. The amplitude is from the baseline to the trough (green lines). The b- wave delay is measured from trough of the a- wave to the peak of the b- wave. The height of the vertical red line is the b- wave amplitude.

actually outside the macula, so therefore these light-adapted ERGs are insensitive to detecting macular disease.

Interpreting ERGs

Usually, ERGs will come with a report detailing the key findings. The key areas to look at are:

- Amplitudes of a-, b- and flicker waves
- Time to peak (a-, b-, flicker peak)
- b-:a- wave amplitude (reduced amplitude indicates inner retinal dysfunction)
- Comparing dark- and light-adapted changes

Using the knowledge we have been over, you can work out that if the DA3 ERG shows a reduced a- wave amplitude but normal b- wave, this suggests a problem with the rod photoreceptors. Where DA3 b- wave is reduced with preserved a- wave, this suggests that the rod bipolar cells are dysfunctional. As DA3 includes a cone element as well, we would need to look at the LA responses as well. As these are exclusively tests of cone function, their normality would mean that the problem is isolated to the rod system. If LA responses showed reduced amplitude, the DA responses will also be affected, but not to as great an extent.

Another exam favourite question is relating to the 30 Hz cone flicker, which is reduced in birdshot disease in particular, and monitoring of this particular ERG represents a way of monitoring the response to treatment in birdshot chorioretinopathy. Below are some examples of illustrative ERG patterns for select conditions that bring together the details we have been over.

Electronegative ERG (Figure 32.5)

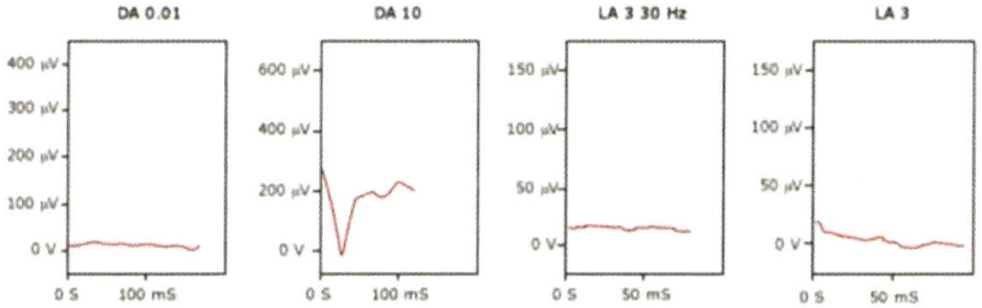

This is an ERG with smaller b- wave than a- wave and can be described in either the dark- or light-adapted state. There is a narrow list of differentials.[1] This can often appear as an exam questions so it is worth knowing the top 5:

- X-linked retinoschisis
- Complete congenital stationary night blindness
- Central retinal artery occlusion
- Birdshot chorioretinopathy
- Melanoma-associated retinopathy
- Autoimmune retinopathy
- Juvenile Batten disease
- Oguchi disease
- Fundus albipunctatus

The ERG in Figure 32.5 shows an electronegative ERG in DA10. This is an example of what a central retinal artery occlusion ERG may look like. The other ERGs are mostly flat or extinguished. This extinguished appearance can also be seen in advanced retinitis pigmentosa.

Rod–Cone Dystrophy ERG (Figure 32.6)

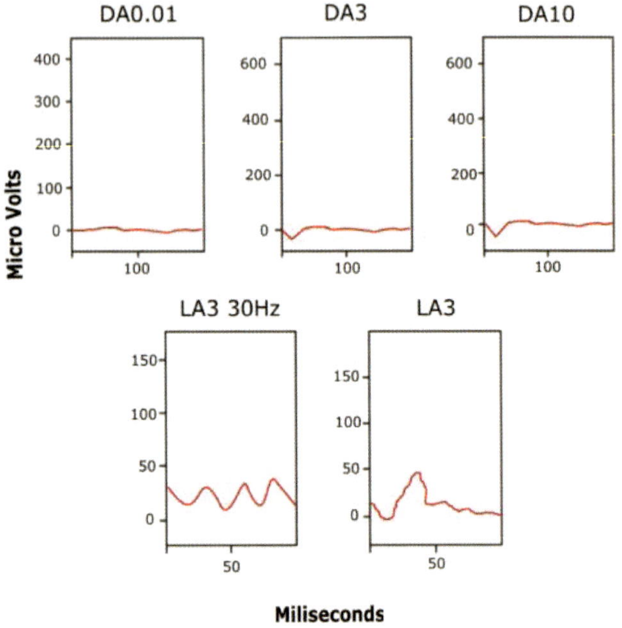

Retinitis pigmentosa is a rod–cone dystrophy (rods affected more than cones), which is reflected in this ERG. You can see the DA responses are nearly completely flat, but there are still some LA responses.

Cone Dystrophy ERG (Figure 32.7)

In this cone dystrophy, all the LA responses are heavily diminished in amplitude whilst the DA responses are all normal. This would represent a less severe cone dystrophy, where it is severe, DA responses would also be affected, though not to the same extent as LA responses.

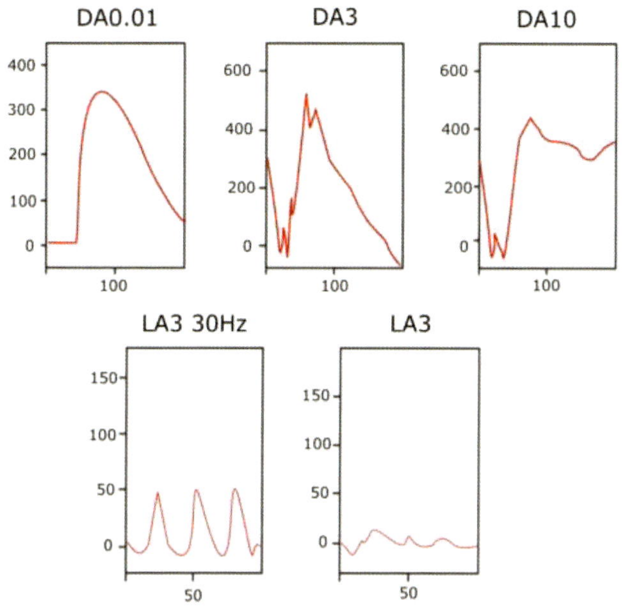

Birdshot Chorioretinopathy ERG (Figure 32.8)

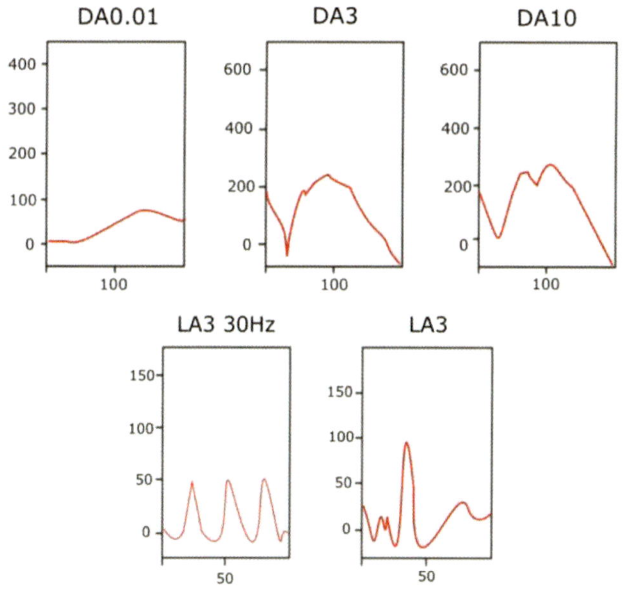

There is evidence of marked reduction in LA amplitudes, including the 30 Hz cone flicker as previously mentioned. There is also general rod system dysfunction as evidenced by the abnormal DA0.01. Note the b- wave is reduced more than the a- wave, leading to a reduced b-:a- ratio, which points towards pathology after phototransduction. In birdshot, inflammatory foci are present in the RPE and result in inner retinal dysfunction that affects both rods and cones. The 30 Hz cone flicker is the most sensitive parameter that is consistently diminished in birdshot cases.

Multifocal ERG

This is more sensitive than a ffERG. It uses a pattern of alternating hexagons to test around 40°–50° of the central retina. It is a measurement of macular function principally.

It produces a waveform with an initial dip (N1) followed by a peak (P1) and then a further dip (N2) (Figure 32.9A), which tests cone responses predominantly. The bipolar cells generate most of the electrical activity. The amplitude of the N1 peak and the delay from the N1 dip to the P1 peak are the main parameters of relevance, in particular the timing provides a better measure of function than amplitude.

Multifocal ERGs are particularly useful for detecting subtle pathology that may cause focal problems in the macula affecting the mid-outer retina. These may mean that full field responses are not initially abnormal. One example is hydroxychloroquine toxicity. Current recommendations from The Royal College of Ophthalmologists' hydroxychloroquine toxicity screening are that multifocal ERG should be performed where there is evidence of a structural defect on OCT or autofluorescence, but no evidence of functional compromise on 10-2 visual field testing. This is because the multifocal ERG will provide a much more sensitive examination of mid-outer retinal function than the 10-2 visual field test (Figure 32.9B).

Multifocal ERGs are only performed by a few tertiary centres in the UK, so you will not be expected to interpret or perform

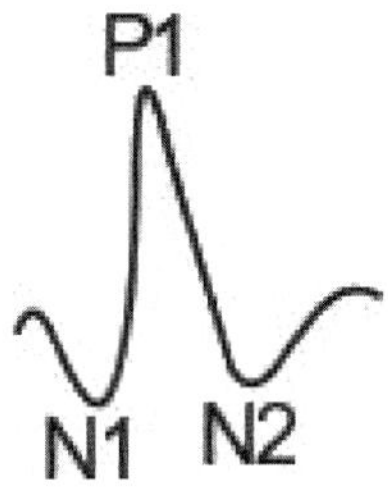

Fig. 32.9A Example mfERG waveform.

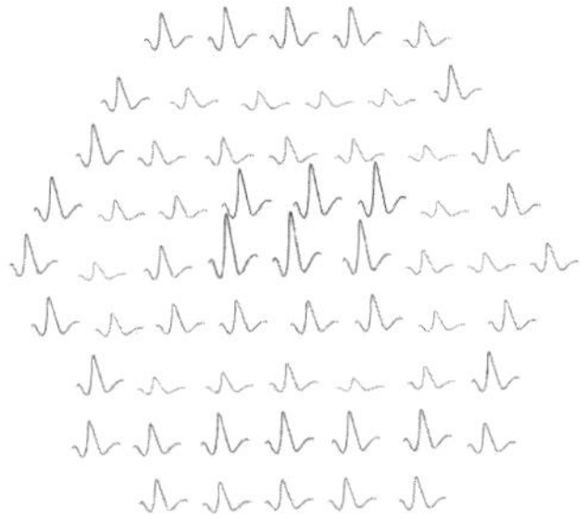

Fig. 32.9B Example of a hydroxychloroquine maculopathy pattern. Early in the disease there may be a bull's eye maculopathy where the central macula is spared but the middle macular function is supressed, as you can see in the diminished waveforms in this mfERG.

these yourself. However, it is useful to be familiar with the principles of the test.

Pattern ERG (pERG)

The pERG uses a reversing checkerboard as shown below (Figure 32.10). For each checkerboard a waveform is produced consisting of an initial trough (N35) then a peak (P50) and a further trough (N95) as shown in Figure 32.11. The checkerboard display is reversed in a room of fixed (low) luminance. The pERG predominantly measures ganglion cell function, with a smaller contribution from photoreceptors. The pERG provides information restricted to the macular region. However, there can be retrograde degeneration of ganglion cells from optic nerve disease (results in reduced P50 height) so the primary

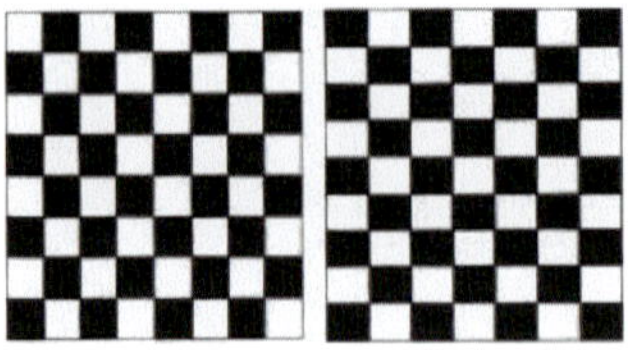

Fig. 32.10 Reversing checkerboard pattern.

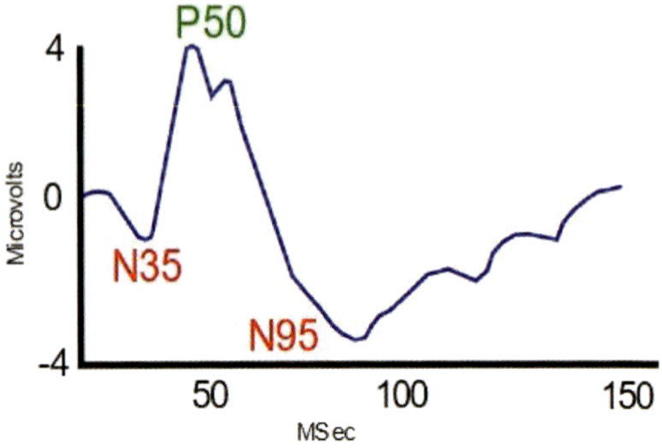

Fig. 32.11 Normal pERG waveform.

pathology may be located outside the macula region. VEPs combined with pERG and ffERG can help localise pathology. Where the ffERG is normal but the pERG is abnormal, it points towards the macula as the source of pathology. Where the VEPs also show abnormality, it means that there is a combination of optic nerve disease with retrograde degeneration of retinal ganglion cells. In cases where the pERG and VEPs are normal but a patient feels they still have vision loss, a non-organic (i.e. functional) visual loss is present.

ELECTRO-OCULOGRAM (EOG)

This is an exam favourite question as the EOG is almost exclusively used in Best's retinal dystrophy. A reduced Arden ratio is the key pathological finding.

The EOG works by measuring the standing potential across the eye. The cornea has a positive polarity relative to the negative polarity of the retina. A positive electrode is attached

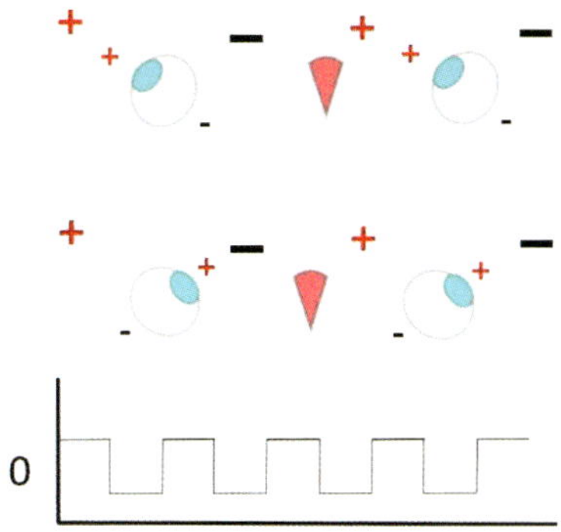

Fig. 32.12 Schematic drawing of EOG. The red cone is the patient's nose. There is a positive and negative electrode on either canthus. The movement of eyes back and forth horizontally will change the charge of each canthal electrode relative to a reference electrode. This produces positive and negative deflections when the voltage is plotted graphically. These peaks and troughs are large in the light and smaller in the dark.

to the skin on one canthus, and a negative electrode to the other. When the eye looks from left to right, the electrodes will register a change in voltage (Figure 32.12).

In the light the potential difference across the RPE rises; in the dark it falls. When performing the EOG, the patient makes horizontal saccades in light conditions and dark conditions. These readings produce a dark trough and light rise. The difference between these two gives the Arden ratio which is usually more than 1.8.

Flash ERGs are normal in Best's disease but the EOG is abnormal. Other photoreceptor disorders can cause abnormal EOGs but will also cause abnormal ERG. Although Best's disease causes a macular lesion, it actually affects the whole RPE, which is measured on EOG, as the standing potential across the whole eye is measured.

VISUAL EVOKED POTENTIALS

VEPs assess the whole visual pathway, from retina to visual cortex. Like the ERG these can be either pattern VEP (pVEP) or flash VEP (fVEP). fVEPs assess the visual pathway response to a bright flash of light. It is useful where there are dense media opacities or children who will not be able to undertake pVEP testing.

Flash VEPs

The waveform (Figure 32.13) does not correspond as neatly to particular anatomical areas as ERGs. N1 and P1 are partly derived from pre-cortical sources. N2 and P2 are from the primary visual cortex. Other peaks, e.g. P3, are possibly extrastriate in origin. Waveforms can also vary considerably with age and between individuals, so the main parameter of interest is the P2 peak at 100 ms which is consistent between individuals. fVEPs are an indicator of a normally functioning central retina and visual pathway beyond.

The VEP can be used in combination with ERGs to investigate the level of maturity of the visual system in infants, provide information about visual potential and localise pathology. The fVEP is however insensitive to central retinal problems, which can be dysfunctional yet produce normal VEPs.

fVEPs are particularly used in cases of childhood albinism. One of the features of this condition is chiasmal misrouting (Figure 32.14), so there is an excessive amount of decussation at the chiasm. pVEPs can still be used to assess chiasmal crossing, but tend to be used in an older age group.

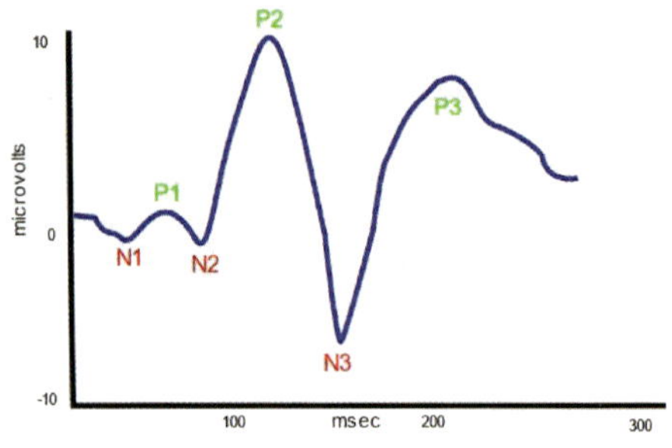

Fig. 32.13 The fVEP waveform.

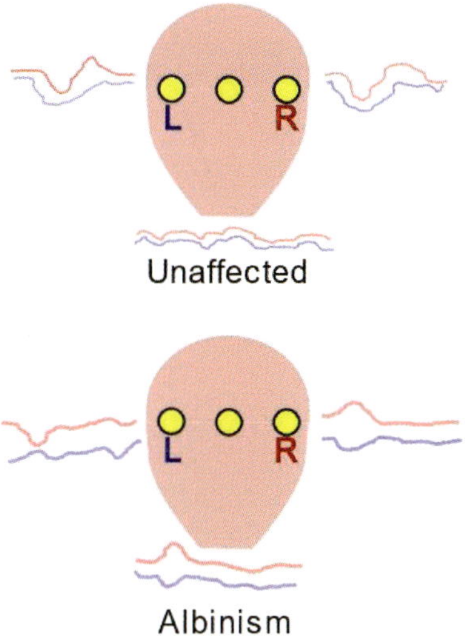

Fig. 32.14 Usually, the peaks and troughs for each electrode should roughly align where there is symmetrical crossing. Where there is asymmetric crossing due to chiasmal misrouting, the peaks of the right electrode correspond with troughs in the reading from the left, which is corroborated in the central reading that is measuring the difference between the two waveforms.

Three occipital electrodes (right, midline and left) are placed to record the signal from either side of the visual cortex. In excessive decussation, a positive waveform in one electrode and a negative in the other is seen due to the more complete crossing. In unaffected individuals, the waveforms should be similar between electrodes. Due to the simple nature of the test, fVEPs can be used in very young children and babies to assess for albinism. Children over 3 years old may be able to undertake pVEP testing.

Pattern VEP

This uses the reverse checkerboard previously described. The pVEP is more sensitive a test than fVEPs, but like fVEP it assesses the whole visual pathway from central retina to visual

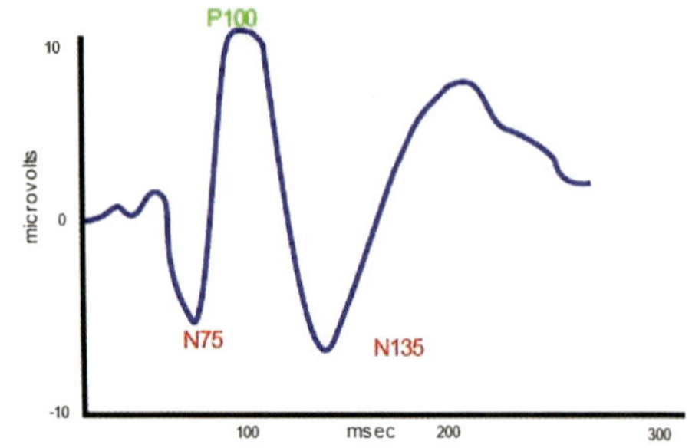

Fig. 32.15 pVEP waveform. The key measurement is the p100.

cortex. It is not sensitive to detecting changes outside central retina. There are two relevant parameters, amplitude and delay of p100. Loss of amplitude indicates axonal atrophy, whereas increased delay is seen in demyelination. Unlike the fVEP, the pVEP can provide some surrogate measure of acuity, by assessing responses as the size of the checkerboard is changed.

CONCLUSIONS

EDT is complex; however, hopefully you can now understand the basics of why certain tests are requested and the relevant anatomy tested by each electrodiagnostic intervention. It is useful to see these tests being performed to get a better idea of the practicalities of how the tests are done. The reports generated by these tests are usually interpreted by specialist neurophysiologists; however, it is useful to be able to understand how the tests relate to clinical queries you may want answered.

Reference

1. Jiang X, Mahroo OA. (2021) Negative electroretinograms: genetic and acquired causes, diagnostic approaches and physiological insights. *Eye* **35**(9): 2419–2437.